EAT TO PR_ _ _

AND CONTROL

DISEASE

COLLECTION

(2 Books in 1)

**Eat to Prevent and Control Disease and
Eat to Prevent and Control Disease Cookbook**

LA FONCEUR

Eb
emerald books

Eb
emerald books

ALSO BY LA FONCEUR

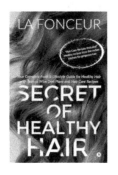

SECRET OF HEALTHY HAIR

If you are seeking a permanent solution to your hair problems, then *Secret of Healthy Hair* is for you! Your complete food & lifestyle guide for healthy hair with season wise diet plans and hair care recipes.

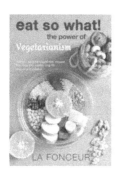

EAT SO WHAT! THE POWER OF VEGETARIANISM

Understand your food scientifically with *Eat So What! The Power Of Vegetarianism*. learn how you can prevent anemia, vitamin b12, and protein deficiency with vegetarian foods naturally without any man-made supplements.

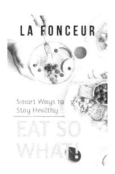

EAT SO WHAT! SMART WAYS TO STAY HEALTHY

Confused about what to eat and what not to eat for health? Clear your confusion with *Eat So What! Smart Ways to Stay Healthy*. This book explains the nutritional value of foods, gives direction on what to eat and gives smart tricks and tips to make life healthier.

CONTENTS

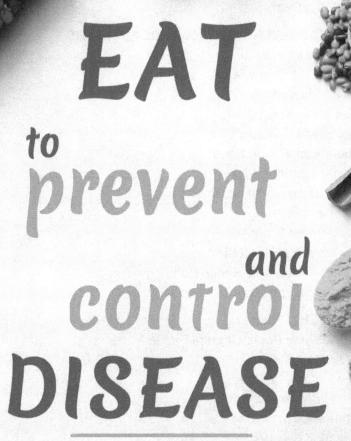

EAT
to
prevent
and
control
DISEASE

**HOW SUPERFOODS CAN HELP YOU LIVE
DISEASE FREE**

LA FONCEUR

EAT

TO **PREVENT**

AND **CONTROL**

DISEASE

How Superfoods Can Help You Live Disease Free

LA FONCEUR

Eb

emerald books

Dear reader,

*The aim of **Eat to Prevent and Control Disease** is to help reduce your dependence on medicines by providing you with in-depth knowledge of common chronic diseases as well as the best food options that prevent and control diseases naturally.*

Eat healthily, live happily!

Master of Pharmacy,

Research Scientist and

Registered Pharmacist

INTRODUCTION

Nowadays, diabetes, high blood pressure, and arthritis have become quite common. One in every family has one of these diseases. People have started considering these diseases as part of life, which is not good. The lifestyle we are leading today - high intake of processed foods, frequent eating out, smoking, and alcohol, there is a 70% chance that you will have either high blood sugar levels or high blood pressure or both by your 50s.

A disease state in the body means your immune system is constantly busy fighting the disease, soon your immune system loses its effectiveness and becomes weak. If another disease strikes, your immune system is unable to fight, this can have life-threatening consequences. It is very important to start as early as in your 20s to take care of your health. Make your body strong enough to fight any disease naturally.

More diseases mean more medicines. Being from a pharmacy background, I can assure you that dependence on medicines is not good. Medicines prescribed in disease have side effects. To reduce side effects, you are often prescribed with another set of medicines that treat the side effects of your primary medications, but they also have side effects, for which again some other medications are required, so basically, this cycle continues. But there is a solution! You can include foods in your diet that have the same effect as your medications. By regular intake of these foods, you can heal your body and increase your immunity to fight disease naturally.

The objective should be to prevent disease, and preparation starts in your 20s. What you eat in your 20s affects your 50s. To prevent a disease, you must have a thorough knowledge of the disease, such as why it happens? How does it affect your body? What exactly does happen in your body in the event of a disease?

What are other health problems that can be caused by a particular disease?

In *Eat to Prevent and Control Disease*, all these topics will be discussed in detail. You will learn about foods that boost your immunity, superfoods that can protect you from diseases, foods that reduce inflammation in your body, and food combinations that you should eat for maximum health benefits.

You will also learn everything about the three most common chronic diseases- diabetes, high blood pressure, and arthritis. To prevent these diseases, which foods and lifestyle options should you avoid, and which ones should you adopt? What should be your strategy to prevent and control these diseases. What are the foods that mimic your medication's mechanism of action and can help lower your blood pressure and sugar levels? What are the key points that you can follow to prevent arthritis and get rid of it? So, get ready for a healthy tomorrow.

1
EAT TO PREVENT DISEASE

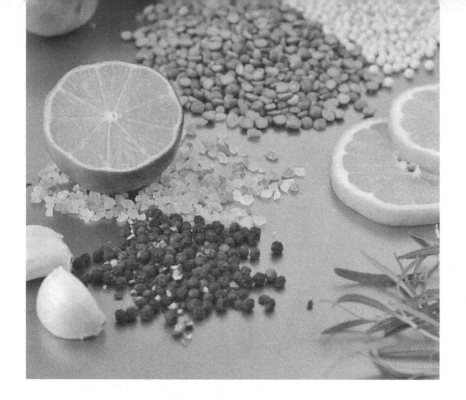

1

ROLE OF FOOD THERAPY IN PREVENTING AND CONTROLLING DISEASE

If you have your blood sugar levels checked for the first time, and your report says that your blood sugar is high, your doctor will not first prescribe you the medicines. Instead, your doctor will give you a three-month time so that you can control your sugar with diet and lifestyle modifications. If the blood sugar is still not controlled, then only you will be prescribed with medicines to control high sugar levels.

You know why? Because medicines treat disease, but they can cause strong side effects. The stronger the drug, the stronger will be its side effects. It doesn't mean you should stop taking medicines without informing your doctor. Never stop your medication without consulting your doctor because some medicines have withdrawal effects, which can even worsen your disease condition if you stop taking them suddenly.

So, what is the solution? The solution lies in good management. You can prevent or manage the disease only when you have comprehensive knowledge about that disease. Everything is on your hand, and you are the commander of your life and your disease condition. With the correct nutrition and healthy lifestyle, you require fewer medicines, shorter therapy duration, and minimum side effects.

When it comes to disease management, there are lots of misconceptions associated with it. Let's first clear these misconceptions:

#1 Misconception
I am young, and I don't have any disease, I have plenty of time to live without worrying. I will worry about diseases when I will hit my 50. Till then, my motto is You Only Live Once.

Actually, you only die once but live every day, so make your every day disease-free. The age of 20 to 40 is your key to make your 50+ years healthy and happy. The way you treat your body between these years, its effect is seen in your old age. These are your sowing years, eat as many healthy foods as you can during these years, and reap the benefits in your 50+ years. Strictly avoid smoking, alcohol, and other drugs that deteriorate your health internally. The harm never visible during your 20s and 30s, but it has life-threatening consequences soon after you hit your 50s or nowadays even in your 40s. Eat junk foods but only to satisfy your taste bud, definitely not to fill your tummy.

#2 Misconception
I am a very health-conscious person, and I believe nature has all the solutions. Although I have been diagnosed with a disease, but I

believe I don't need medication. I can heal myself naturally with healthy food and a good lifestyle.

If you have been diagnosed with a disease means the harm has unknowingly already been done. Keep in mind medicines are not the enemy, just they are not a natural food. Sole dependence on medicines is not good; at the same time, completely abandoning medicines when your body needs them is also not right. No doubt, healthy foods, and healthy lifestyle choices can heal you much faster, but you definitely need medication to treat a disease. With healthy foods, you can heal yourself faster, and your body recovers more quickly, so you need a shorter course of therapy that simply means lesser side effects.

#3 Misconception
Last time when I had these symptoms, my doctor prescribed these medicines. Now again, I feel the same problem, I should take the same medicines as the doctor had prescribed me last time.

Avoid self-medication. In a condition of reoccurrence of any disease, medicines may be the same, but with different doses. Don't be a doctor yourself. Self-medication may result in an overdose, which can lead to toxicity and other life-threatening consequences. Seek advice from your doctor every time you are not feeling well and ask him/her directly if it is safe to take the same medication again when the symptoms occur. Always ask your doctor about what should be the diet in managing your disease? Ask your pharmacist if there is any food that you should avoid while taking the prescribed medicine.

#4 Misconception
I was on medication, and my condition has improved. Although my doctor had prescribed me a 3-month course of medicines, I was feeling fine, so after two months, I stopped taking the medicines.

This is never advised. Maybe with your healthy diet and lifestyle, you have recovered faster than others, but you should never leave your medication course in between without consulting your doctor. Even if your symptoms are relieved with initial medications, you need the full course to treat the disease completely. Otherwise, it will reoccur, and as it has not been treated in the initial stage, it will reoccur with more severeness. Abruptly discontinuing some medicines produce withdrawal effects in the body and worsen the disease condition. Instead of quitting your medicines, you should inform your doctor about your improvement. Your doctor will gradually reduce the dose of the same medication and complete the course sooner than before, or he will advise you to complete the full course depending upon your disease type and your condition.

#5 Misconception
I am taking medicine for my illness, and medicine is doing its job. It will cure me, I don't need to worry about nutrition and all.

Food and lifestyle play a huge role in managing any disease. If your diet is not healthy and your lifestyle is also not good, then your condition may worsen despite regular medication. Foods that boost immunity prepare your body to fight the disease and heal your body. A healthy lifestyle removes the burden from your body; hence your body can completely focus on treating the disease.

#6 Misconception
Some diseases like diabetes, high blood pressure, arthritis, etc. come naturally with age. You cannot escape from these diseases. Every other person I know has one of these diseases, so this is pretty normal at my age.

It may be common but indeed not normal. This is the biggest myth that some diseases naturally come with age. With age, our body becomes a little weaker, but most of these diseases are the result of our poor diet and poor lifestyle. It's time to stop letting these diseases become part of your life and build your body with healthy foods and a healthy lifestyle in such a way that these diseases never even touch you, and if you already have these diseases, then they can be controlled.

DISEASE MANAGEMENT

What is a disease?

A disease is a condition of disturbances in the normal structure or function of your body. When something goes wrong with the normal function of your body, your body gives signals in the form of signs and symptoms that something is going wrong inside the body. This is where your responsibility begins. With proper medication, healthy foods, and healthy lifestyle, you can prevent and treat disease.

Disease is mainly managed with medications and foods and lifestyle modifications. Let's understand the role of each.

ROLE OF MEDICATIONS

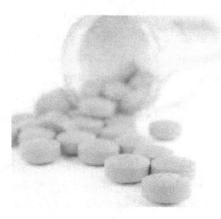

Prescribed medications play a vital role in the treatment. Generally, medicines work in three ways:

1. To reduce symptoms like pain, nausea, and fever.
2. To treat the disease.
3. To reduce or treat the side effects arising due to the use of medicines in curing the disease. Such as antacids are usually prescribed with high dose medications as these medications can cause acidity in the body.

It is important to take the medicines at the same time every day. Medicines take their time (onset time) to show their effect on the body. Taking medicines at the same time every day ensures that its active ingredient will be available in the body uniformly throughout the treatment.

ROLE OF LIFESTYLE CHOICES

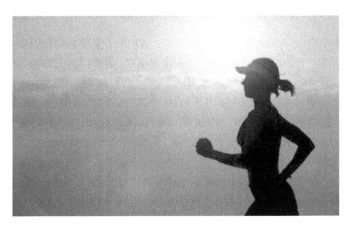

Poor lifestyle choices give a burden to your body. In simple terms, these are the inducer of many diseases. Unhealthy lifestyle choices weaken your body, lower your immunity, and make you susceptible to many diseases.

Example of unhealthy lifestyle choices:
- Stress
- Smoking
- Alcohol
- Unhygienic habits
- Inadequate sleep

When it comes to poor lifestyle choices, you may have found plenty of discussions about smoking, alcohol, and inadequate sleep, but we often take other poor lifestyle choices such as stress and unhygienic habits lightly.

Stress is a key contributor to many diseases. When you are under stress, your body releases the stress hormone cortisol, which causes your heart to pump faster and raises your blood pressure. After the stressful time has passed, your body releases lower amounts of cortisol. Your heart and blood pressure return to normal. But if you are under constant stress, the consistently high levels of cortisol in your body can cause many health problems. Take out at least 2 hours for yourself every day, do nothing during this time, just relax. Just two stress-free hours in a day gives your body enough time to normalize all its functions and systems.

Unhygienic habits such as not washing your hands before eating and after using the washroom, and touching an open wound allow germs to enter the body. As a result, your immune system keeps busy fighting these germs and with time immune system weakens. When your immune system becomes weak, it can't protect you from major and serious diseases. So, don't stress out your immune system. Already there is so much pollution in the environment with which your immune system fights daily, so do not give it more burden. Maintain good hygiene and keep your immune system healthy. Whenever you come from outside, first wash your hands with soap water. This habit will protect you from many diseases. Also, 5-Second rule is a big myth. Even a brief exposure of the floor can contaminate your food with E. coli, salmonella, and other bacteria in under five seconds.

What should be your focus points to prevent disease?
If you keep your immune system and digestive system healthy, you greatly lower your risk of diseases.

Avoid Immune weakening lifestyle choices
- Stress
- Smoking
- Drinking Alcohol
- Consuming narcotics such as Cannabis

Adapt the immune-boosting lifestyle choices
- 7-8 hours of sleep
- Washing your hands frequently

- Expose yourself to early morning sunlight
- Yoga
- Taking a walk after lunch and dinner

Avoid immune weakening foods

- Trans fats
- Processed foods
- Canned foods
- Refined carbohydrates
- Foods high in sugar

Add immune-boosting foods in your diet

- Foods rich in vitamin C
- Foods high in zinc
- Foods that have anti-inflammatory effects

ROLE OF FOODS

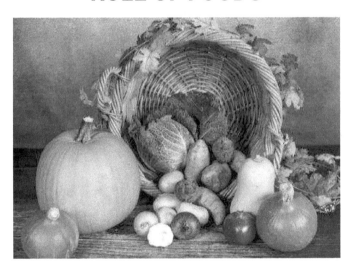

Foods play a massive role in every stage of disease management. These roles include:

1. To prevent the disease.
2. To shorten the therapy period.
3. To control the disease.
4. To prevent the reoccurrence of the disease.

Body is nature's product, and your body loves natural things like food. Plant-based healthy foods can prevent various diseases and autoimmune disorders and help build your body strong enough to fight off any disease. Plant-based healthy foods heal your body, reduce your dependency on medicines, and add disease-free years to your life.

Why food therapy is the best therapy?

Medicines work on the disturbance that has been arisen in your body dues to disease, while foods work on the root cause and strengthen your body to fight with the disease naturally. Moreover, foods have no side effects. A simple rule is to include vegetables and fruits of every color in your diet; it will protect you from countless diseases.

We are so concerned about avoiding unhealthy foods that it has become quite stressful now. The more you try to run away from them, the more you crave. If you do not eat unhealthy foods, but your diet lacks essential nutrients, then there is no health benefit of avoiding unhealthy foods. To stay healthy, incorporating healthy foods into your diet is more important than just avoiding unhealthy foods. It is time to focus on what you should eat, not what you should not eat. Do not modify your diet for weight loss; instead, balance your diet for a healthy and disease-free life.

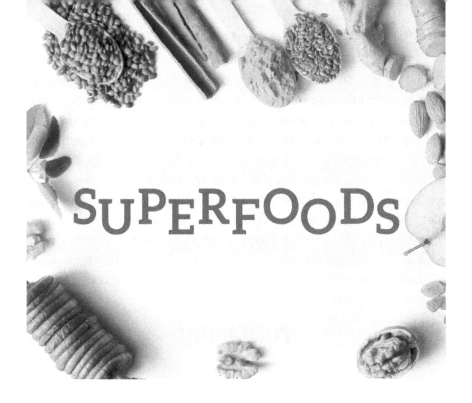

2

10 SUPERFOODS YOU MUST EAT EVERY DAY TO LIVE DISEASE-FREE

Foods can protect you from many diseases and can improve your disease condition. Superfoods are foods that are highly dense in nutrients. A food is considered as a superfood when it not only can protect or treat a single disease, but its regular consumption can protect you against many diseases at a time. Eating just superfoods and avoiding other foods doesn't guaranty you a disease-free life. But eating superfoods every day definitely reduces the risk of developing the disease manifold. This is because superfoods contain active chemical compounds that are antioxidant and anti-inflammatory, and inhibit oxidative stress by killing free radicals and reduce inflammation in the body.

Oxidative stress and inflammation are the leading causes of cancer, arthritis, diabetes, and many such chronic diseases. You can prevent these diseases by eating superfoods every day. Do not look at superfoods as medicines that you only need until your condition improves. See them as lifelong friends; They are here to do good for you, so you must keep their company throughout life. I am listing top superfoods that you must include in your everyday diet. But to stay disease-free, you should also avoid eating processed foods, canned foods, fried items, salt, and other well-known health deteriorators. Here are superfoods that have medicinal properties and can reduce your dependency on medicines. Let's meet our lifelong food friends:

TURMERIC

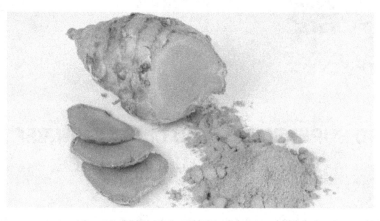

Turmeric deserves to be at the top of the superfoods list. Turmeric has scientifically proven health benefits. The credit goes to curcumin, the active compound of turmeric. Curcumin gives the bright yellow color to turmeric and has many medicinal properties. It is a potent anti-inflammatory, antioxidant, antibacterial, antiviral, and antifungal agent. These properties play an important role in keeping your body strong enough from inside to prevent most of the disease.

Inflammation is good for the body as it helps heal an injury or fights infection, but our today's food and lifestyle cause inflammation in the body at a dangerous level. Chronic inflammation is one of the reasons for almost every disease, including arthritis, heart disease, Alzheimer's disease, depression, cancer, and other degenerative conditions. Curcumin has potent anti-inflammatory property which protects you from many diseases. Lower levels of Brain-Derived Neurotrophic Factor (BDNF) is associated with Alzheimer's and depression. Turmeric boosts the levels of BDNF and very effective in preventing and treating depression and Alzheimer's disease.

Turmeric helps prevent and control a variety of cancer types, including prostate, breast, colorectal, and pancreatic cancers. It helps stop the growth of tumor cells.

Due to its antibacterial and antiviral property, curcumin might help fight off infection and a variety of viruses, including herpes and viral flu. So, next time when you get a viral fever, add one tablespoon of turmeric powder in milk, boil for two minutes, and drink it before bed. It will heal you faster.

Turmeric protects cells from the damage caused by free radicals. Unhealthy foods like foods high in saturated fats, sugar as well as poor lifestyle choices such as drinking alcohol contribute to free radicals, which is associated with tissue damage. Free radicals can cause damage to cells of DNA, proteins, and cell membranes, by pairing with their electrons through the oxidation process. These are responsible for aging and other health complications. Turmeric has a high content of polyphenols, flavonoids, tannins, and ascorbic acid; these all are the natural antioxidants and help protect cells from the damage caused by free radicals.

How to consume turmeric?
Eat fresh turmeric in the winter season. Grate it and add in your morning tea. In other seasons, use turmeric powder in cooking and have hot turmeric milk at night before bed. Turmeric is warm in nature, so don't overeat it in summer, you may get mouth ulcer.

Who should avoid turmeric?

No one. It can consume by anyone. Eat black pepper with turmeric; it increases curcumin absorption in the body. However, if you are taking blood-thinning medicines like warfarin, you should limit your turmeric consumption because turmeric purifies the blood and thins the blood.

How much turmeric should I eat in a day?

You should aim to get 500mg-1000mg of curcumin in a day, which is equivalent to one tablespoon of freshly ground turmeric or one tablespoon of turmeric powder. Avoid supplements rather than go for fresh or powdered turmeric.

FENUGREEK LEAVES AND SEEDS

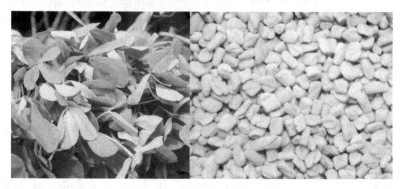

Fenugreek leaves and seeds have a wide range of nutrients that provide numerous health benefits. They are packed with iron, vitamins, biotin, choline, flavonoids, and fibers. The high antioxidant flavonoid content in fenugreek seeds can reduce pain and inflammation and improve arthritis conditions. Fenugreek leaves and seeds are high in soluble fiber, which helps lower blood sugar and decreases cholesterol levels. The fiber in fenugreek slows down the digestion and absorption of carbohydrates and is very effective in controlling diabetes. High blood cholesterol levels increase your risk of heart diseases. The soluble fiber in fenugreek gets attached to cholesterol particles and takes them out from the body, thus decreasing the cholesterol levels in the body and reduces blood pressure. This reduces the risk of developing heart complications and improves heart health.

Also, fenugreek seeds are effective in the treatment of hair loss, male impotence, and other types of sexual dysfunction.

How much fenugreek should I consume in a day?
One teaspoon of fenugreek seeds in a day for six months to see the result. Aim to eat fresh fenugreek leaves every day or every alternate day in the winter season.

What is the best way to consume fenugreek?
Soak one teaspoon of fenugreek seeds in a glass of water overnight. Next morning, chew the fenugreek seeds and swallow them with a full glass of water (in which seeds were soaked). Make fresh fenugreek leaves salad or sauté them in mustard oil, add garlic to enhance the taste.

Who should avoid fenugreek?
If you are on medication of diabetes or hypertension, don't start taking fenugreek in high amount without consulting your doctor and pharmacist. Fenugreek may perform similar functions as your diabetes and BP medications. So taking both may lower blood glucose and blood pressure below the safe range. Because of that, the dose of your medicines might need to be changed.

FLAX SEEDS

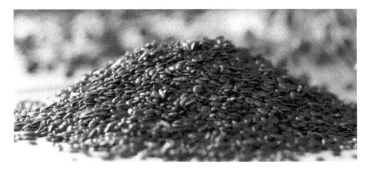

Flax seeds are probably the healthiest among all the seeds. They have got the reputation of superfood because they are packed with cancer-fighting polyphenols lignans, alpha-linolenic acid

(ALA), and fibers. Flax seeds contain approximately 100 times more lignans than any other plant foods, which helps in protecting against breast cancer, colon cancer, and prostate cancer. They are one of the best sources of an omega-3 fatty called acid alpha-linolenic acid (ALA). Due to their high omega-3 content, they help reduce the risk of heart disease, stroke, and diabetes through their anti-inflammatory action. Omega-3 fatty acid alpha-linolenic acids, along with lignans, block the release of pro-inflammatory agents and reduce inflammation in the body. The anti-cancer property of flax seeds is due to their lignans content; they suppress the growth, size, and spread of cancer cells by blocking enzymes that are involved in hormone metabolism.

How much flax seeds should I eat in a day?
One tablespoon (10g-15g) of flax seeds in a day.

What is the best way to eat flax seeds?
Dry roast and grind them. Add the ground flax seeds in chapati and tortilla dough.

Who should avoid flax seeds?
There are no side effects reported till date, so it is safe to eat flax seeds for all. Always remember moderation is the key. Consuming too much flax seeds with too little water can worsen constipation and may lead to an intestinal blockage, so take flax seeds with plenty of water to prevent this from happening.

SWEET POTATOES

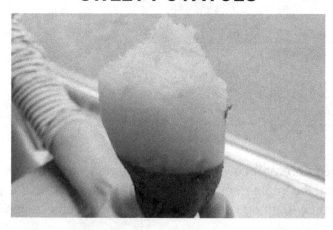

Sweet potatoes are one of the best sources of beta carotene that converts into vitamin A in the body and promote eye health as well as boost immunity. Beta carotene functions as a potent antioxidant that reduces cell damage and helps prevent the free radical damage that is associated with cancer. The higher fiber content of sweet potatoes prevents constipation and promotes a well-functioning digestive tract. The presence of anthocyanin pigments in sweet potatoes, particularly in purple-fleshed sweet potatoes, helps in preventing chronic inflammation in the body.

Sweet potatoes are rich in both magnesium and potassium, both of which are essential in lowering blood pressure and reduce the risk of cardiovascular diseases.

Higher fiber and magnesium content of sweet potatoes may decrease diabetes risk. Moreover, sweet potatoes help to regulate the blood sugar levels, especially in people with diabetes; its high insoluble fibers content promotes insulin sensitivity. Unlike other starchy foods, sweet potatoes have a low glycemic index. They release sugar into the bloodstream slowly and steady, which aids in controlling the blood sugar levels of individuals.

How many sweet potatoes should I eat in a day?
One medium sweet potato in a day is enough to meet your daily recommended vitamin A intake.

What is the best way to cook sweet potatoes?
To get the most nutrition from your sweet potatoes, don't peel them, simply wash, and scrub well before cooking. They can be boiled, steamed, and baked. Steamed or boiled sweet potatoes have more healthy benefits than baked sweet potatoes because baking releases the sugar inside the sweet potato, which may increase blood glucose levels.

Who should avoid eating sweet potatoes?
People who have existing kidney stones or are at high risk of developing them or those who are on dialysis should avoid sweet potatoes. It is because sweet potatoes are high in potassium, and

when you have kidney disease, your kidneys cannot remove extra potassium, and too much potassium can stay in your blood.

COW'S MILK

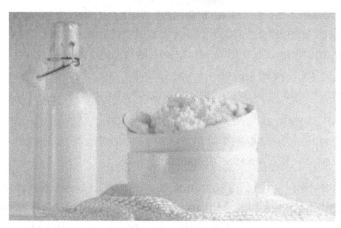

The reason why you should drink milk every day is because cow's milk is a complete food means it contains every nutrient that you need in a day for a healthy body. Cow's milk is packed with protein, calcium, potassium, vitamin A, B vitamins, and phosphorous. When you feel hungry, have a glass of cow's milk, it's enough to give you energy for the next 2 -3 hours.

Let's see why milk is so good for your health:

Amino acids are compounds that combine to make proteins. Your body needs nine essential amino acids through food to maintain normal functioning. Not all protein sources are considered as a high-quality complete protein because not all protein-rich foods contain all nine essential amino acids. Milk is a rich source of protein, mainly casein (80%) and whey (20%). Both are complete protein because both contain all nine essential amino acids that are required for body to maintain good health.

Milk is an excellent source of calcium, which is necessary to build healthy bones and teeth and to maintain bone mass. The presence of vitamin D in milk increases the absorption of calcium in the body. Calcium with vitamin D can protect you from osteoporosis. Magnesium and potassium in milk support proper kidney and heart function and can help prevent hypertension and heart diseases.

Milk is a complete package; you can get all essential nutrients in a single, convenient source. If you are thinking of switching to vegan, keep in mind that it is hard to have all milk's nutrients in a single vegan food source. Most of the vegan sources are fortified means extra nutrients are manually added to them, and these nutrients are not naturally present in them, so basically, these are not natural sources. Also, when you switch to vegan, you need supplements to reach daily vitamins and minerals need of the body, which is an effective way but again, not the natural way. Anything which is not natural is not advisable to depend on for a long time.

Milk products that you should add in your diet:
Cow's milk (best for health), low-fat yogurt, buttermilk, cottage cheese, and cow's milk's ghee.

Milk products that you should avoid:
Heavy cream, processed cheese, and whole-fat dairy products.

How much milk and milk products should I consume in a day?
250 ml cow's milk + 2-3 milk products (yogurt, cottage cheese).

Who should avoid milk?
If you are lactose intolerant, you should avoid milk. Another alternative is lactose-free cow's milk, which contains all the nutrients of milk, but it's free from lactose. Lactose-free cow's milk is made by adding the enzyme lactase to cow's milk, which breaks down the lactose into glucose and makes it lactose-free and can easily be digested by lactose-intolerant people.

Limit your dairy consumption in the wet season. Consuming too much dairy can aggravate gastric problems, cause nausea, diarrhea, and stomach pains, even though if you are not lactose intolerant. So, moderation is the key.

If you have a cough, limit your milk and milk product consumption. Avoid taking milk at night. Milk doesn't increase the production of phlegm, but it can make your existing phlegm thicker and may irritate your throat and aggravate a cough.

RAW GARLIC

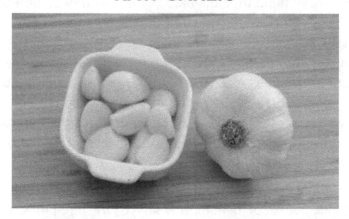

Garlic is an adaptogen which means it stabilizes and maintains a steady internal environment in the body, in response to environmental changes. It ensures the optimal functioning of the body, including the regulation of body temperature, blood sugar, blood pressure, pH balance, and functioning of the immune system. This is the reason why initially garlic had used for medicinal purposes only. Most of the potent medicinal properties of garlic are due to the allicin, a sulfur compound that gives pungent smell to the garlic. The thing with allicin is that it only releases when you crush or cut the garlic. Allicin is very unstable, which means you need to use it immediately after you cut garlic. The allicin in raw crushed garlic is destroyed by heat. So, for health benefits, eat fresh raw garlic.

Also, garlic protects against bowel and stomach cancers. It is scientifically proven that the sulfur components of garlic alter the biological behavior of tumors, tumor microenvironments, and precancerous cells. Garlic decreases cancer risk, particularly cancers of the gastrointestinal tract.

Garlic is known to contain natural antioxidants that can eliminate low-density lipoprotein (LDL) cholesterol from the body and help protect against heart disease by thinning the blood and improve blood circulation. Garlic reduces both systolic and diastolic blood pressure by increasing the nitric oxide production in the body, which helps smooth muscles to relax and widen the blood vessels.

The antibacterial and antifungal properties of garlic help fight infections and boost the function of the immune system. So basically, this vegetable (yes, it's vegetable, not an herb or spice) can actually protect you from many diseases. It's time to add RAW garlic in your diet!

How should I take garlic?
Eat one clove of freshly crushed raw garlic every morning on an empty stomach. Don't eat more than one clove of fresh raw garlic at a time. Don't keep garlic in the mouth for too long; it may cause burn. Eat plenty of garlic (raw and cooked) in winter, add them in soup or spring roll. Limit garlic consumption in the summer season, too much of garlic in summer, may result in acne and ulcer due to its heat-producing nature.

When should I avoid garlic?
If you have ulcers, colitis, acid reflux, or heartburn problem, limit your garlic consumption.

How much garlic is enough for health benefits?
One clove of raw garlic (crushed) on an empty stomach every day is enough. If you experience heat, ulcer or acid reflux, then instead of daily, eat it twice or thrice a week.

SPROUTS

Sprouts are affordable, safe, and easily grown nutrient-dense superfood. Sprouting can increase nutrition up to 100 times than raw legumes and vegetables.

For those who have difficulty digesting certain foods, sprouting is a better option for them. The reason is sprouting increases the proteolytic enzymes content of the food that break down starches into simpler carbohydrates, proteins into amino acids, and fats into fatty acids. So, your digestive system need not break them, which makes these nutrients more bioavailable and easily digestible.

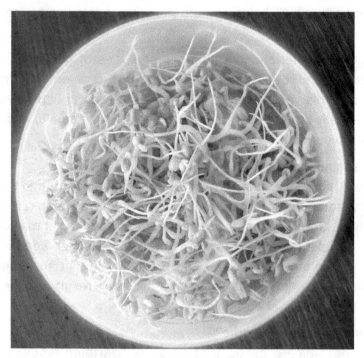

Why is sprouting beneficial for you? Because sprouting increases the nutrition value of legumes and vegetables, it removes enzyme inhibitors and unlocked healthy compounds. The increased bioavailability of high levels of vitamins, minerals, amino acids, essential fatty acids, and antioxidants increases the alkalinity of your body. Raising pH (to an alkaline state) increases the ability of your immune system to prevent disease.

Grow sprouts at your home to reduce your exposure to pesticides, food additives, and other chemicals. There are so many different sprouts varieties you can try, including mung bean, black chickpeas, lentils, wheat sprouts, alfalfa, radish seeds, and broccoli.

How many sprouts should I eat in a day?

Eat a bowl of different varieties of sprouts in a day. You don't need to eat the same sprouts every day, keep them rotating, eat every sprout on alternate or every three days, but try to have a bowl of sprouts every day.

What is the best way to eat sprouts?

Eating them raw will keep all the nutrients locked. To make them tangy, add finely chopped cucumbers, onions, tomatoes, fresh-squeezed lemon juice, black salt, and black pepper.

Who should avoid eating sprouts?

In case you are going for store-bought sprouts (which I would not recommend at all), don't eat them raw. Cook them thoroughly until steaming hot throughout to reduce the risk of food poisoning from Salmonella, Listeria, or E. coli. Store-bought sprouts can be contaminated anywhere along the journey from farm to table. People with weakened immune systems should not eat any variety of raw or lightly-cooked sprouts; it may result in food poisoning.

SPINACH

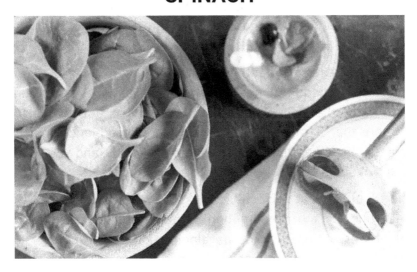

Spinach is called a superfood because of its anti-inflammatory and antioxidant properties. It is packed with iron, vitamin k, protein, calcium, magnesium, and potassium that protect your body from a wide range of diseases. Spinach is a significant source of vitamin K, which is an important factor in wound healing and bone health. Spinach is rich in carotenoids that are beneficial antioxidants that boost your immune system. It contains three different types of carotenoids: beta carotenoid, lutein, and zeaxanthin.

Beta carotenoid converts into vitamin A in the body and has a vital role in maintaining healthy vision, healthy immune system, and healthy reproduction system. Lutein and zeaxanthin function as a light filter, protecting your eye tissues from UV rays of sunlight.

The high levels of potassium in spinach, along with folate, relaxes the blood vessels and lower your blood pressure. Spinach also helps the body make nitric oxide, a natural vasodilator which further lowers blood pressure.

Often people who have type 2 diabetes have low levels of magnesium. Spinach is very low in calories and has a low glycemic index. Additionally, it is rich in magnesium, which helps to lower blood sugar and can even protect you from type 2 diabetes.

What is the best way of eating spinach?
The more you cook spinach, the more it will lose its nutrients. Either sauté the spinach or blanch the spinach, but don't blanch for more than 1 minute. Add lemon juice while blanching, it will increase the absorption of nutrients in your body, and you will get the full health benefit.

Who should not eat spinach?
Limit your spinach consumption if you have kidneys stone or if you are at a high risk of developing kidney stones because spinach is high in both calcium and oxalates that can cause kidney stones.

If you are taking blood-thinning medication, do let your doctor and pharmacist know about your spinach consumption. Spinach is high in vitamin K that promotes blood clotting and can decrease the effectiveness of your blood-thinning medication such as warfarin.

DRY FRUITS

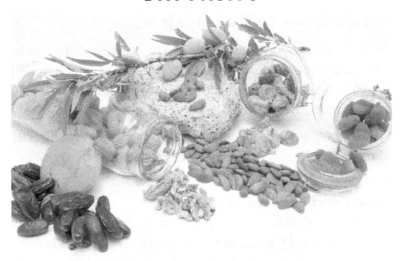

You must have heard this 1000 times that you should eat nuts every day! But do you follow it? If not, then it's time to start eating nuts every day! Eating dry fruits every day helps promote overall well-being and ensures a healthy, disease-free long life. Nuts contain heart-friendly monounsaturated and polyunsaturated fats, and antioxidants like flavonoids and vitamin E. Research suggests that high consumption of nuts, including peanuts, is associated with two to three times reduced risk of breast cancer.

Dry fruits are high in fiber and magnesium, which help to stabilize blood sugar and insulin levels. Dry fruits lower the risk of developing type 2 diabetes.

Dates are loaded with iron and potassium and yet contain little sodium, which helps maintain normal blood pressure and keeps the risk of a stroke in check.

Dried figs are a good source of calcium. Figs keep bodily systems like the endocrine, immune, respiratory, digestive, and reproductive system in check.

Almonds are an excellent source of vitamin E, protein, and monounsaturated fats. They promote weight loss by reducing hunger and keeping you full for a longer period. The healthy fats and antioxidants of almond lower blood pressure and cholesterol levels and also lower the blood sugar levels.

Walnut kernels don't just look like a brain, but they actually contain brain-boosting polyphenolic compounds like omega-3 fatty acids. Polyphenols are considered critical brain food and prevent cognitive disorders.

Cashew nuts are rich in zinc, which boost immunity and prevent male pattern baldness and prostate enlargement by blocking the creation of Dihydrotestosterone (DHT).

How many dry fruits should I eat in a day?
Eat a handful of different dry fruits every day, including almond, walnut, cashew nuts, pistachio, dates, raisins, and figs. Frequency matters, so it is important to eat them every day even if the quantity is less than a handful.

What is the best way to eat dry fruits?
Nuts contain phytic acid that reduces the nutrition value of nuts by lowering absorption, so the best way to remove phytic acid is soaking. Soak a handful of dry fruits in water overnight and eat them the next morning.

Who should avoid eating dry fruits?
You should eat plenty of dry fruits in winter but limit your dry fruits consumption in the summer season. Nuts produce heat in the body, while it is beneficial in winter to keep you warm; in summer, it can give you acne, ulcer, and acidity.

BASIL LEAVES

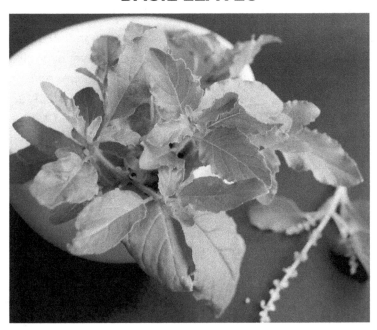

Holy basil or tulsi is a superfood because it is an immunomodulator and adaptogen. It lowers blood sugar levels, cholesterol, and triglycerides.

Stress increases your risk of developing or worsens conditions like hypertension, diabetes, heart disease, Alzheimer's disease, depression, obesity, and gastrointestinal problems. Adaptogen with anti-inflammatory properties of basil helps you to reduce stress, anxiety, depression, and very effective in preventing and treating cognitive disorders, including amnesia and dementia. The neuroprotective, anti-stress, and anti-inflammatory activities of basil enhance memory and improve brain function. For this reason, basil considers as a natural memory tonic.

Regular consumption of basil leaves can prevent viral infections. Research confirms that holy basil has an immunomodulatory effect; it increases the percentage of T-helper cells as well as NK-cells (Natural killer cells), which are the components of the adaptive immune system and innate immune system, respectively. These cells help eliminate pathogens by preventing their growth and help fight viral infections.

Research shows basil leaves are as effective in lowering blood glucose as antidiabetic drugs. Basil leaves have hypoglycemic properties, which lower blood sugar levels and improve insulin sensitivity. If you have prediabetes or type 2 diabetes, the essential oil of basil helps cut down cholesterol and triglyceride levels, which is a persistent risk factor for type 2 diabetes.

How much basil should I consume in a day?
Start your day by chewing two to three fresh basil leaves.

What is the best way to eat basil leaves?
Add 2-3 fresh basil leaves in your morning green tea. You don't need much expertise in growing basil at your home.

Who should avoid eating basil leaves?
Limit your basil consumption if you are taking medications like acetaminophen or paracetamol (pain reliever). If you are consuming plenty of basil leaves and taking paracetamol, they both work together and tend to affect the functioning of your liver.

CONCLUSION

Now that you know the foods that can naturally protect you from diseases, should you just opt for their dietary supplement? Not at all. Supplements are never recommended in place of natural foods. This is because the supplements contain ingredients that have strong biological effects in the body. Their dose may interfere with medications you may already be taking, which can sometimes have harmful consequences. Taking too much of some supplements can have life-threatening consequences. You should include various natural foods in your diet, not human-made foods, so supplements are a big no in replacing superfoods.

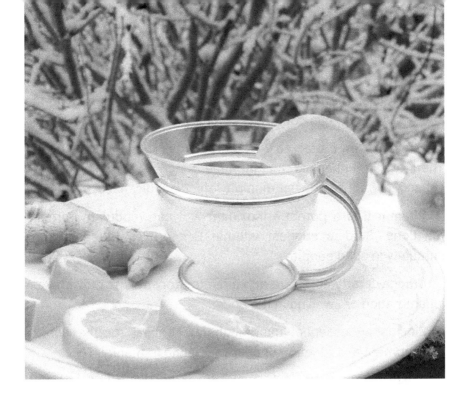

3

10 POWER FOODS TO BOOST YOUR IMMUNITY

Keeping your immune system healthy, directly means protecting yourself from many diseases. In winter, cold and flu are quite common but have you ever thought why few people get flu while others not. The reason is their immunity. Some people have a naturally strong immune system, while others have weak. No matter whether your immunity is naturally strong or weak, you can definitely boost your immunity with some power foods. This will not only make your winter flu-free, but it will also protect you from many diseases.

When it comes to immunity, the five major nutrients that need to be taken into consideration are as follow:

Vitamin C is the most crucial nutrient for boosting your immunity. Vitamin C supports various cellular functions of the immune system, thus contributes to immune defense.

Vitamin A promotes as well as regulates the immune system. Therefore, it enhances the immune function and provides an enhanced defense against multiple infectious diseases.

Vitamin E is a potent antioxidant and can modulate immune functions. Studies suggest vitamin E improves the decreased immunity in aged people.

Omega-3 fatty acids are anti-inflammatory means they prevent inflammation or swelling in the body.

Zinc is an essential mineral that is crucial for the normal development and function of cells mediating immunity.

These five nutrients are crucial for maintaining and boosting immunity. A deficiency in any of these nutrients may weaken your immune system. Eating foods rich in zinc, omega-3, vitamin A, C, and E, help you build a stronger immune system. Let's see which power foods contain an abundance of these crucial nutrients.

Below are the 10 power foods to boost your immunity, so, start adding them in your diet for a disease-free, healthier life:

1. Citrus fruits

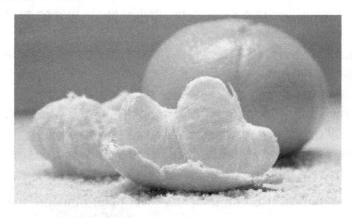

If you think of immunity, the first name that comes in your mind is vitamin C! and why not? Vitamin C is actually the best nutrient when it comes to immunity. It protects against immune system deficiencies, skin wrinkling, cardiovascular disease, eye disease, etc. Vitamin C increases the production of white blood cells, which are an essential part of the immune system. These are the key to fight infections by killing bacteria and viruses that invade the body. Citrus fruits such as lemon, tangerine, orange, and grapefruit are high in Vitamin C.

Citrus fruits are a natural antioxidant that boosts the immune system. These have antiviral and antibacterial properties that prevent infections, bacterial growth, and relieves nausea.

Squeeze one medium lemon in one glass of warm water (250 ml) and drink it every morning. You need vitamin C daily for continued health, so make a habit of taking lemon water instead of plain water every morning.

2. Turmeric

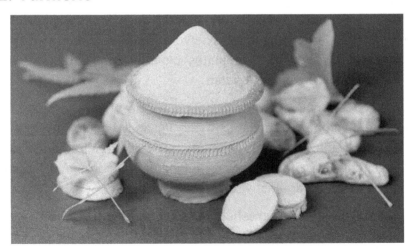

This bright yellow spice is a natural immunomodulator that boosts your immunity. Curcumin, the active compound of turmeric has many scientifically-proven health benefits. Curcumin is a potent antioxidant and has anti-inflammatory effects. Turmeric not only boost your immunity but also very effective in treating both rheumatoid arthritis and osteoarthritis. Add one tablespoon of turmeric powder in hot milk (250 ml) and drink it every night just before bed and see the magic yourself.

3. Garlic

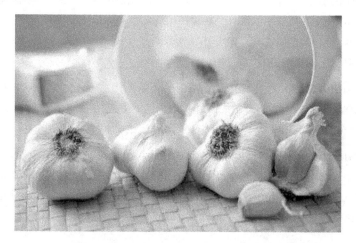

Garlic is an adaptogen, which means it helps the body to adapt varied environmental and psychological stresses and supports all the major systems, such as the nervous system, immune system, and hormonal system. It regulates blood sugar; if they are too high, it will lower it and vice-versa.

Garlic contains active compound allicin that improves the immune cells' ability to fight off the flu and reduces the risk of infection. Garlic also has anti-inflammatory, antibacterial, and antiviral properties that help in inhibiting the growth of some bacteria and fight against viral infections.

Taking one clove of crushed garlic on an empty stomach every day not only boosts your immunity but also normalizes all major systems in your body. If your body is already acidic or warm in nature, limit the consumption to 3 times a week.

4. Ginger

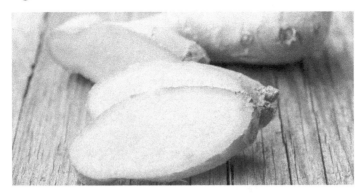

The bioactive substance gingerol in the ginger root has anti-inflammatory and anti-fungal properties. It helps in lowering the risk of infections and relieving a sore throat. It also helps fight viruses such as rhinoviruses, human respiratory syncytial virus (HRSV), which cause colds, and many respiratory infections. Ginger is a strong antioxidant, it naturally boosts your immunity. Drinking ginger tea every morning in the winter season keeps you warm and saves you from cold and flu.

5. Flax seeds

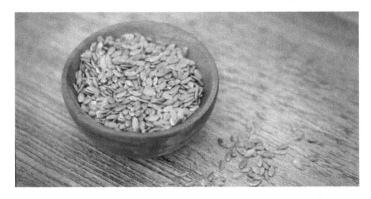

Flax seeds are rich in Omega-3 fats that help protect your body against bacteria and viruses, improving your immunity. Flax seeds contain the highest concentrations of dietary lignans that help protect against cancer by blocking the growth and spread of tumor cells. These are also a great source of iron that ensures your immune system gets required oxygen to fight infection. The omega-3 fatty acids of flax seeds fight inflammation in the body and prevent inflammatory diseases such as rheumatoid arthritis, psoriasis, and lupus.

6. Red and green bell peppers

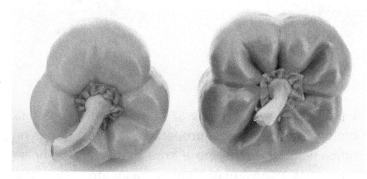

If you think orange or lemon is the richest source of vitamin C, then here is the surprise, bell peppers contain twice as much vitamin C as any citrus fruit. They are also a rich source of beta carotene, which converts into vitamin A in your body. The high content of both vitamin C and vitamin A in bell peppers enhance your immune function and provide enhanced defense against multiple infectious diseases. Vitamin A is an anti-inflammation vitamin that helps in treating and preventing arthritis and contact dermatitis. Eat cooked bell peppers because cooking increases vitamin C content in bell peppers.

7. Cashews

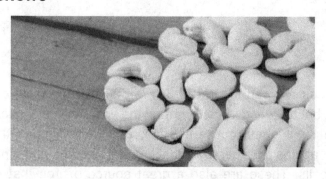

Cashews are a great source of zinc and copper. Zinc plays an important role in the production of immune cells and antioxidant enzymes that help fight disease and infection. Cashews have antioxidant effects that help your body fight off oxidative damage. Cashews speed up the healing of wounds as they are rich in vitamin K. Vitamin E of cashews help decrease inflammation in your body. Pregnant women must eat cashews as they help with the growth and development of the baby.

8. Papaya

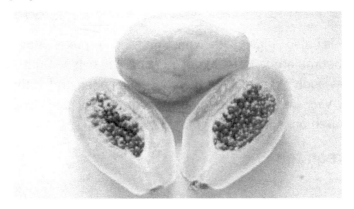

Papaya has antioxidant and immunostimulant effects that reduce oxidative stress and improve immune functions. Papayas also contain potent antioxidants known as carotenoids — particularly lycopene. Carotenoids are converted into vitamin A in the body and help regulate the immune system. Papaya is also a great source of vitamin B, C, and K and known as an excellent immunity booster. It slows down the aging process and helps your skin look more youthful and supple. One medium-sized papaya can fulfill your daily requirement of vitamin A.

9. Yogurt

It is said that the healthier your gut is, the better will be your immunity. Yogurt is the best probiotic. Yogurt contains lactobacillus, a probiotic, or good bacteria that help keep your gut healthy, also gives your immune system a boost.

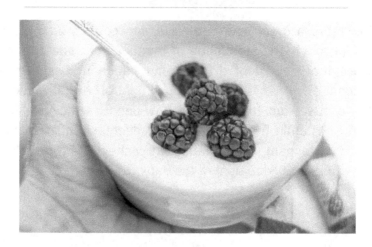

Yogurt is also high with vitamins and protein. Due to the immunostimulatory effects of yogurt, it helps fight against diseases such as infection, GI disorders, cancer, and asthma. It is actually very beneficial for older people. Go for plain yogurt, not the flavored ones, and eat it with your lunch.

10. Green tea

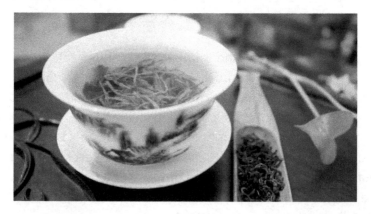

The list is incomplete without the mention of green tea. The higher concentration of polyphenols and flavonoids, the two powerful antioxidants, make green tea a gem for boosting your immunity. These antioxidants kill the free radicals in the body and increase your longevity.

Free radicals are the by-products of the process where cells use oxygen to generate energy in the body. At low or moderate levels, free radicals are harmless, but at high concentrations, they cause oxidative stress, a deleterious process that can damage all cell structures. Oxidative stress plays a crucial role in the development of arthritis, autoimmune disorders, cancer, aging, cardiovascular and neurodegenerative diseases.

The powerful antioxidants in green tea kill these free radicals and help in fighting illnesses, like common cold, arthritis, aging, and cancer. Start drinking green tea if you have not started yet!

CONCLUSION

These foods definitely boost your immunity, but to keep your immune system healthy, it is also important to have a healthy lifestyle that includes getting sufficient sleep, doing yoga, taking a morning walk, and managing your stress. Definitely, there are dietary supplements available in the market to boost your immunity, but their effects are limited. One good thing about going natural is, it comes with all benefits with no side effects. Most of the immune booster foods also enhance your skin and hair health, so it's a win-win situation.

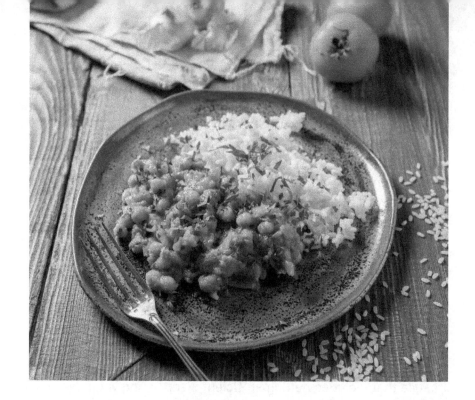

4

10 NUTRIENT COMBINATIONS YOU SHOULD EAT FOR MAXIMUM HEALTH BENEFITS

Nutrients need to adequately absorbed into your body to provide health benefits. Some nutrients are eliminated faster from your body without being absorbed, and you don't get their health benefits. Various factors affect the absorption of nutrients. Foods require a favorable environment inside your body and the presence of certain vitamins and minerals to get absorbed. If foods don't get absorbed in your body, you don't get the health benefits. Fortunately, you can enhance the absorption of food by pairing it with other food that can provide an environment required for their absorption and prevent their metabolism, making the nutrient more available in the blood to get absorbed. Eating these foods together ensures that you get maximum health benefits.

Below are 10 nutrient combinations that you should eat for maximum health benefits.

1. Vitamin C + Iron

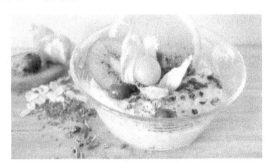

Iron is an essential nutrient required for blood production. Hemoglobin of red blood cells comprises about 70 percent of iron. Hemoglobin transfers oxygen through your blood from the lungs to the tissues. Deficiency in iron may cause iron-deficiency anemia that can lead to heart problems. You may become deficient in iron if you are eating too little iron-rich foods, or the iron is not getting absorbed properly in the body. When you eat vitamin C with iron, it increases the stability and solubility of iron by binding with them. Once iron becomes more soluble, it allows the body to more readily absorb the iron through the mucus membranes of the intestine.

Food combinations that you should eat for better iron absorption:
1. Lemon juice + Spinach
   Add lemon juice when blanching the spinach, it will retain the green color of spinach as well as increase the iron absorption.
2. Lemon juice + Sprouts
3. Tomatoes + Lentils
4. Orange + Oatmeal
5. Tomatoes + Beetroot

2. Vitamin D + Calcium

Calcium and vitamin D both are very important for your bone health. Not only your bones but your heart, muscles, and nerves also need calcium to function properly. You must have noticed that the prescribed calcium tablets always come in a combination of vitamin D. There is a solid reason behind it. Vitamin D is the fat-soluble nutrient that increases the absorption of calcium in the intestine. Calcium, along with vitamin D, not only can protect you against osteoporosis and bone disease. This combination can even protect against diabetes, high blood pressure, and cancer.

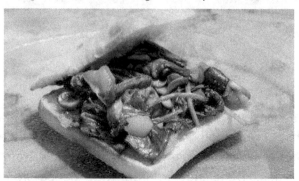

Food combinations that you should eat for better calcium absorption:
1. Expose your skin to sunlight for 10 to 15 mins in the morning after that drink a glass of milk.
2. Mushrooms + Soybeans
3. Yogurt + Nuts
4. Mushrooms + Dark leafy greens
5. Sour cream + Broccoli

3. Turmeric + Black pepper

Turmeric has health benefits due to its active compound curcumin. The problem with curcumin is its poor absorption in the body. Additionally, curcumin is rapidly metabolized in the body that leads to its rapid elimination from the body. As a result, you could be missing out on its health benefits. By combining turmeric and black pepper, you can increase curcumin bioavailability. Black pepper has active ingredient piperine that protects curcumin from the digestive enzymes. It slows down the breakdown of curcumin. As a result, curcumin remains in the bloodstream for a longer period. It, therefore, boosts the absorption of curcumin by multiple times, making it more readily available to be used by the body.

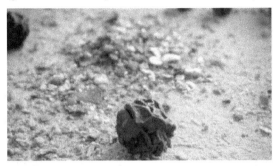

4. Zinc + Vitamin A

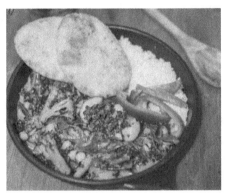

Vitamin A is not only crucial for protecting against night blindness, but it also promotes healthy growth and development and has a very critical role in enhancing immune function. Absorption of vitamin A is hugely affected by zinc availability in the body. Zinc plays a vital role in the absorption, transporting, and utilization of vitamin A in the body. When your body is deficient in zinc, it affects the movability of vitamin A from the liver to body tissues. Zinc also regulates the conversion of retinol (vitamin A) to retinal that requires the action of a zinc-dependent enzyme. So, if you eat vitamin A-rich foods together with zinc-rich foods, you will get the maximum health benefits of vitamin A.

Food combinations that you should eat for better vitamin A absorption:
1. Cashew nuts + Carrot cake

2. Legumes + Spinach

3. Dry fruits + Mango milkshake

4. Swiss cheese + Sweet potato

5. Oats + Papaya

5. Green tea + Lemon

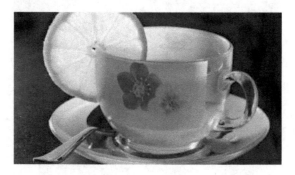

Green tea is loaded with catechins which are the polyphenols that have potent antioxidative, anti-inflammatory, and antibacterial activity. Catechins improve blood pressure, blood sugar levels, prevent cell damage and very effective in preventing cancer. The catechins of green tea are relatively unstable in the intestine. Vitamin C rich foods such as citrus fruits increase the amount of catechins available for the body to absorb. Vitamin C interacts with catechins to prevent their degradation in the intestines. As a result, more catechins are available to absorbed in the body. So, make sure to add lemon juice in your green tea because when you add lemon in your green tea, it increases catechins absorption by more than five times.

6. Phytic acid + Water

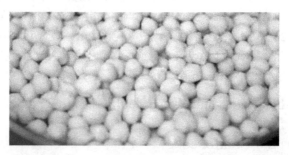

Plant-based foods such as whole grains, legumes, and nuts contain phytic acid that binds with minerals such as iron, zinc, calcium, and manganese and prevents their absorption in the body. When phytic acid binds with these minerals, it forms phytates, and our bodies do not have any enzymes that can break down phytates to release these minerals. So, you don't get the full health benefits of these minerals. Fortunately, the simple solution to this problem is soaking! Soaking in water allows the phytic acids to leach onto the water. You should soak phytic acid-containing foods in water overnight (or for at least 3-4 hours). It will increase the bioavailability of the minerals and decrease gastrointestinal distress.

Foods that you should soak for better absorption:
1. Nuts (Almond, peanuts, walnuts, and others)
2. Legumes (kidney beans, chickpeas, and peas)
3. Rice
4. Wheat bran
5. Sesame

7. Tomato + Olive oil

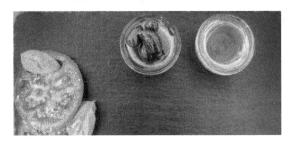

Lycopene is the main carotenoid in tomatoes. The antioxidant lycopene of tomatoes is responsible for reducing the risk of heart disease and certain types of cancer. Lycopene is a fat-soluble compound, which means it is better absorbed in the presence of healthy fat. Eating tomatoes cooked in olive oil greatly increase the absorption of lycopene and protect your cells against free radicals, which play a role in aging, heart disease, cancer, and other diseases.

8. Folate + Vitamin B12

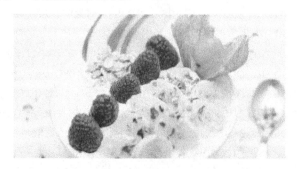

Folate (Folic acid or vitamin B9), when taken alone, can mask the symptoms of vitamin B12 deficiency. The problem is that without symptoms, you will not know that you are deficient in vitamin B12. This can delay the diagnosis, and there could be a risk of developing nerve damage. Because of this reason, these vitamins are often taken together. Moreover, folate works closely with vitamin B12 to make red blood cells and to help iron function properly in the body. Folate and vitamin B12 together (along with vitamin B6) help lower homocysteine levels. Study shows high levels of homocysteine (an amino acid) are associated with the development of coronary artery disease, leading to heart attacks and strokes. If you eat folate and vitamin B12 rich foods together, you will never get deficient in folate or vitamin B12, and you will never get depressed because these two vitamins, when eaten together, enhance the immune function and mood.

Folate and vitamin B12 food combinations that you should eat for maximum health benefits:
1. Yogurt + Banana
2. Shiitake mushrooms + Dark leafy greens
3. Milk + Nuts
4. Yogurt + cooked Okra (Ladyfinger)
5. Whey + Lentils

Whey is the by-product of cottage cheese-making. It is the liquid remaining after milk has been curdled and strained. Cook lentils in whey instead of plain water.

9. Rice + Beans (complete protein)

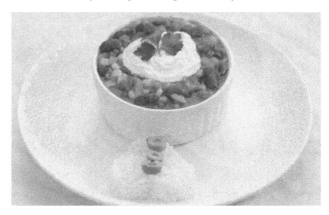

The human body needs nine amino acids, which are essential means you need to get them through food. A complete protein means a food source of protein that contains an adequate amount of each of the nine essential amino acids. Not all protein sources are a complete protein, especially vegetarian protein sources. That doesn't mean being a vegetarian, you will miss out on amino acids. When you eat correct food combinations, you can get all the essential amino acids. The best example is rice and beans. Together, rice and beans form a complete protein because when eaten together, they provide all nine essential amino acids necessary in the human diet.

Beans are rich in lysine but missing an amino acid known as methionine. Rice has high levels of methionine but doesn't have enough amino acid lysine. When rice and beans (such as kidney beans and chickpeas) are consumed together, each provides the amino acid that the other lacks, making it a high-quality protein. Here are some more high protein food combinations.

Food combinations that you should eat to get complete protein:
1. Kidney beans + Rice
2. Green peas + Lentils
3. Corn + Mixed beans
4. Red lentils + Brown rice
5. Cabbage + Wheat

10. Vitamins A, D, E and K + Healthy fats

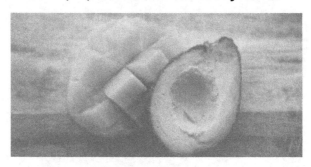

Vitamin A, D, E, and K all are fat-soluble vitamins. These fat-soluble vitamins require the availability of fat to absorb properly in the body. Your body can't absorb them effectively without eating some fat at the same time. Some examples of foods containing fat-soluble vitamins are mango, red bell peppers, sweet potato, and most of the colored vegetables (vitamin A), milk and milk products (Vitamin D), almonds, peanuts, sunflower seeds (vitamin E) and leafy greens like spinach, kale, cauliflower (Vitamin K).

Food combinations that you should eat for better absorption of fat-soluble vitamins:
1. Almond milkshake
2. Nuts roasted in cow's ghee
3. Spinach + Mustard oil
4. Mango + Avocado
5. Nuts + Flaxseeds

CONCLUSION

It is not very hard to eat the food combinations mentioned above. Some of the above food combinations you might already be eating, some combinations might be new to you. It's time to do some experiments with your taste bud. If you come up with a new dish while combining these nutrients, do let me know. I would love to try it too.

2

DISEASE: PREVENTION AND CONTROL

Diabetes

Hypertension

Arthritis

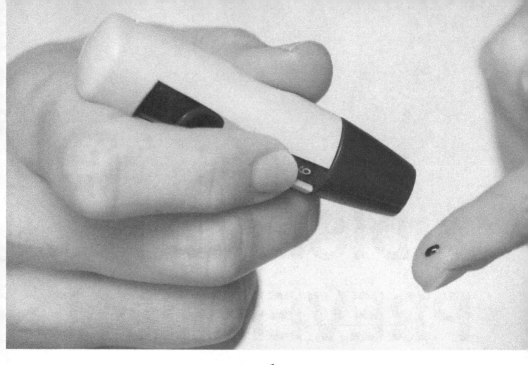

1

DIABETES

1.1

EVERYTHING YOU NEED TO KNOW ABOUT DIABETES

Diabetes is probably the most common chronic disease; 1 in 11 of the world's adult population is living with diabetes. It's like a slow poison. It slowly affects the other part of your body and a major cause of kidney failure, blindness, and heart attacks. The worrying part is people don't take diabetes seriously. The younger generation is not well educated about it, and affected people are highly dependent upon medicines, giving less effort on diet and exercise front. Diabetes doesn't come with age, but it comes with a bad lifestyle and diet deficient in healthy nutrients. If you have type 2 diabetes, you don't need to live with it; diabetes is reversible. Early diagnosis, a healthy diet, physical activity, and medications can help you reverse diabetes. If you have diabetes for a long time and you are on high dose medications, your aim should not be just to avoid sugary foods. You should aim to eat foods that mimic the action of your anti-diabetic drugs and exhibit similar effects in the body and also have no side effects. Regular screening of diabetes complications can help you prevent and treat complications before they become severe.

Here are some dangerous facts about diabetes that no one talks about:

- According to the International diabetes federation, diabetes caused 4.2 million deaths in 2019.
- 374 million people are at increased risk of developing type 2 diabetes, according to IDF.
- According to WHO, diabetes is a major cause of kidney failure, heart attacks, stroke, and blindness.
- Diabetes was the seventh leading cause of death in 2016, according to WHO.

Don't just accept diabetes as a new normal; it may be common but not normal. Let's prevent and control diabetes through natural ways. But for that, first, you need to have thorough knowledge about every aspect of diabetes so that with a little help from health professionals (who can guide you at every step where you will have confusion), you can prevent and control diabetes without medicines.

What is diabetes?

Diabetes is a chronic disease, it occurs either when the body does not produce insulin or does not effectively use the insulin it produces. Insulin is a hormone that helps the body use sugar for energy. Hyperglycemia is the medical term for high blood sugar (glucose) levels. It is a common effect of uncontrolled diabetes. Over time, hyperglycemia leads to severe damage to many of the body's systems, especially the nerves and blood vessels.

TYPES OF DIABETES

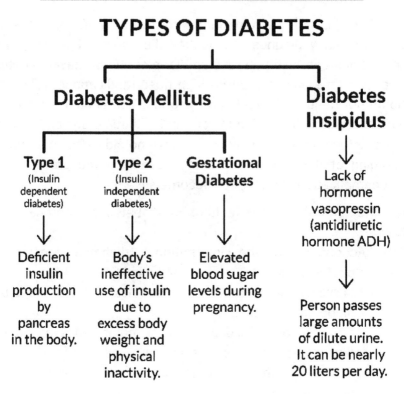

©La Fonceur

DIABETES INSIPIDUS

People with diabetes insipidus have normal blood glucose levels. The only similarity between diabetes mellitus and diabetes insipidus is excessive urination. Diabetes insipidus occurs when kidneys cannot balance fluid in the body. It happens due to some damage in the pituitary gland, which releases the anti-diuretic hormone (ADH), also known as vasopressin. ADH or vasopressin enables the kidneys to retain water in the body. In the absence of vasopressin, kidneys excrete too much water. This causes frequent and excessive urination and can lead to dehydration.

DIABETES MELLITUS

Diabetes mellitus, or simply diabetes, is a disorder that is characterized by abnormally high blood sugar (glucose) levels because the body does not have enough insulin to meet its needs. It is caused either because the body doesn't produce enough insulin or because the body is ineffective in using insulin. In diabetes, urination and thirst are increased and damages the nerves and tiny blood vessels that cause health complications, especially in the kidneys and eyes.

What happens in your body in diabetes?
When you eat food containing carbohydrates, your body breaks them down into sugar (glucose) and send that to your bloodstream. The rise in glucose triggers the pancreas to release insulin into the bloodstream. Insulin signals muscle, liver, and fat cells to take in glucose from the blood. These cells then convert glucose into energy or store it for later use. In diabetes mellitus, your body doesn't use insulin as it should, which results in too much glucose in your blood.

Type 1 diabetes (Insulin-dependent diabetes)

Type 1 diabetes is an autoimmune condition in which the pancreas cannot produce insulin. Typically, the immune system protects your body against the attack of bacteria and viruses by fighting against them. An autoimmune condition is a condition in which your immune system mistakenly attacks your body's cells. In type 1 diabetes, the immune system destroys the beta cells of the pancreas that produce insulin, making the pancreas unable to produce insulin.

Insulin is a hormone that regulates the blood sugar levels in your body. In the absence of insulin, your body can't use or store glucose for energy. The glucose stays in your blood, and your blood sugar or blood glucose levels become too high (hyperglycemia). Persistent high glucose levels result in diabetes and can lead to complications affecting your kidneys, nerves, eyes, and heart. A person who has type 1 diabetes requires daily insulin injections to control blood glucose. The condition usually appears in children and young people, so it used to be called juvenile diabetes.

Type 2 diabetes (Insulin-independent diabetes)

Type 2 diabetes is the most common form of diabetes that primarily occurs due to obesity and lack of exercise. It is characterized by high blood sugar (hyperglycemia) and insulin resistance.

Insulin resistance means your pancreas is releasing insulin as it should, but the cells in your muscles, fat, and liver start resisting the signal given by insulin to take glucose out of the bloodstream for making energy. This results in too much glucose in your blood, known as prediabetes.

In a person with prediabetes, the pancreas works increasingly hard to release enough insulin to overcome the body's resistance and to keep blood sugar levels down. Over time, the pancreas' ability to release insulin begins to decrease, which leads to the development of type 2 diabetes.

Reason for Insulin resistance

The driving forces behind insulin resistance are excess body weight, too much fat in the abdominal area, and a sedentary lifestyle, while genetics and aging also play a role in developing insulin resistance.

GESTATIONAL DIABETES

Gestational diabetes is a condition in which your blood glucose levels become high during pregnancy. Body goes through different changes during pregnancy, such as weight gain and changes in hormones, which affects the body's cells' ability to respond to insulin effectively. Most of the time pancreas can produce enough insulin to overcome insulin resistance, but some pregnant women cannot produce enough insulin and develop gestational diabetes. Mostly, gestational diabetes goes away soon after delivery. Women who develop gestational diabetes during pregnancy are at higher risk of developing type 2 diabetes later in life.

Here is everything about diabetes mellitus that you need to know to prevent and control it:

SYMPTOMS OF DIABETES

Excessive urination (polyuria): To get rid of excess glucose, kidney makes more urine than usual. Daily urine output can be more than 3 liters a day compared to the normal urine output about 1 to 2 liters.

Excessive thirst (polydipsia): Too much glucose forces kidneys to work overtime. Kidneys pull water from tissues to make more urine to help pass the extra glucose from your body, which makes you dehydrated. This usually makes you feel very thirsty.

Fatigue: Because the body's cells do not get enough glucose to make energy.

Weight loss (in Type I diabetes): Because of dehydration caused by excessive urination and loss of calories from the sugar that couldn't be used as energy.

Constant hunger: Because the body can't convert the food you eat into energy.

Blurred vision: High blood sugar causes body water to be pulled into the lens inside the eye, causing it to swell.

WHY IS DIABETES DANGEROUS?

Uncontrolled diabetes can lead to potential health complications, including:

Retinopathy (Eyes damage): High blood sugar levels can weaken and damage the small blood vessels of the retina, which can cause visual disturbance and can even lead to blindness.

Neuropathy (Nerve damage): Constant high blood sugar can damage nerves that typically results in numbness, weakness, tingling, and burning or pain, usually in the hands and feet (diabetic foot).

Nephropathy (kidney damage): Over time, diabetes can damage the small blood vessels in the kidneys, which can lead to kidney failure, and the person may require dialysis or a kidney transplant.

Ketoacidosis (mostly in Type 1 diabetes): When there isn't enough insulin in the body to convert glucose into energy, your body starts breaking down fat for energy. This process produces a build-up of acidic substances called ketones to dangerous levels in the body, eventually leading to ketoacidosis.

Heart disease: Over time, the high blood sugar levels can damage the blood vessels that maintain the heart function, causing them to become stiff and hard. A high-fat diet can cause a build-up of fats and cholesterol on the inside of these blood vessels, which can restrict blood flow. This condition is known as atherosclerosis. Atherosclerosis conditions can reduce blood flow to the heart muscles (which causes angina) and brain (which causes stroke) or can damage the heart muscle, which can result in a heart attack.

DIABETES: PREVENTION AND CONTROL

Diabetes condition can be effectively managed by
Diet
Medication
Exercise
Before going further, let's clear some terms associated with diabetes:

Glycemic index
You must have heard about low glycemic foods and high glycemic foods, but what is exactly the glycemic index?

The Glycemic index helps you differentiate between good carbohydrates and bad carbohydrates for diabetes. Not all carbohydrates are the same. Type of carbohydrates like complex carbohydrates takes longer to break down into glucose and slowly absorbed and metabolized that cause a slower rise in blood sugar. This type of carbohydrates doesn't give you a sudden spike of sugar levels and considered as good carbohydrates. These are categorized as low-glycemic foods; they help maintain good glucose control. Foods that have the glycemic value 55 or less are good for diabetes—for example, whole grains and beans.

Simple carbohydrates such as sugar and highly processed and refined carbohydrates such as pastries and cakes are considered as high glycemic foods. They speedily break down into glucose and quickly absorbed, causing a rapid rise in blood sugar. Repeated spikes in blood sugar lead to an increased risk for type 2 diabetes.

Hypoglycemia

Hypoglycemia condition is often caused by diabetes treatment. Hypoglycemia is the opposite of hyperglycemia. It is a condition in which your blood sugar levels are lower than normal. Certain diabetes medicines or too much insulin may cause your blood sugar levels to drop too low. It is a reversible condition and can be treated by consuming high-sugar foods such as fruit juice or honey. If you are on diabetes medication, you should pay attention to hypoglycemia symptoms, which include confusion, shakiness, and dizziness. If left untreated, hypoglycemia can get worse and can even cause seizures, coma, and death. Always keep glucose tablets with you in case you experience hypoglycemia.

ROLE OF MEDICATIONS IN DIABETES

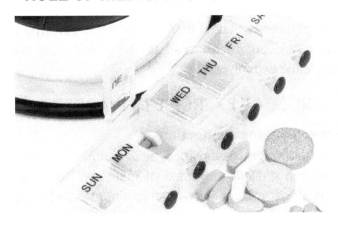

How do diabetes medicines work?

Your most common and first choice of drug in diabetes (metformin) doesn't stimulate insulin secretion by beta cells in the pancreas; instead, it enhances the ability of your tissues to take glucose out of the bloodstream and convert it into energy, especially in muscles. Additionally, it lowers the production of glucose by the liver. It is a drug of choice because it doesn't cause weight gain and hypoglycemia. The common side effect of metformin is diarrhea. Don't just stop taking your medicine because of diarrhea; instead, eat yogurt, beans, an apple, or a banana (not more than one banana in a day) to prevent diarrhea. Make sure to drink plenty of water to prevent dehydration caused by diarrhea.

Another class of drugs (sulfonylureas), reduces high blood sugar by increasing insulin secretion by beta cells in the pancreas. Additionally, it increases cells' sensitivity to insulin, which increases the efficiency of the body's cells to take out glucose from the bloodstream. It also increases the availability of insulin in blood by reducing the degradation of insulin in the liver. The side effects of this class of drugs are weight gain and hypoglycemia. It is very important to keep an eye on your hypoglycemia symptoms, which include shakiness, sweating, dizziness, confusion, irritability, and loss of consciousness. Severe hypoglycemia can potentially lead to coma. Take glucose tablets (total 15g or ask your doctor for exact amount) or foods high in glucose like one tablespoon of honey or sugar or 3-4 raisins to treat hypoglycemia immediately. Ask your doctor to adjust the dose of your medicines if you experience hypoglycemia.

ROLE OF EXERCISE IN DIABETES

Obesity and diabetes connection

Obesity is a common reason for type 2 diabetes. Just by losing weight, you can prevent the onset of diabetes. If you are in the prediabetes stage, you can even reverse diabetes by losing weight, and by including hypoglycemic and weight-loss-friendly foods in your diet.

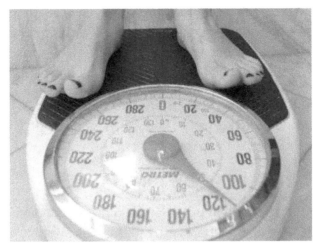

Excess fat may contribute to insulin resistance. It is because when your fat cells that store extra fat become too large, they stop storing fat. Additional fat starts storing in muscles, liver, and pancreas, making these organs resistant to insulin, and they stop responding to the signal given by insulin to take glucose. Moreover, fat cells decrease the secretion of adiponectin, a protein hormone that helps in the breakdown of fat. In simple terms, adiponectin is your fat-burning hormone. High adiponectin levels can protect you against insulin resistance, diabetes, and heart disease. The more you lose weight, the higher your adiponectin levels.

How can weight loss prevent the onset of diabetes?

In type 2 diabetes, insulin production decreases over a sustained period, and the process is rather slow in comparison to type 1 diabetes. It is possible that a strict diet and exercise regime, leading to weight loss, and may delay or even prevent the onset of diabetes. The key is to diagnose the diabetes condition before beta cells function deteriorates.

After the age of 40, you should get your sugar levels tested every year for early diagnosis of high blood sugar levels. If you are overweight, losing weight is your first and most crucial step. It will not only save you from diabetes but can protect you against many diseases. You don't need to lose weight in a short time. Start eating diabetes-friendly foods and start with moderate exercise, soon your body will get habitual of your new diet and exercise regime. It should not be your short-term goal but a new lifestyle.

Ideal weight target to prevent insulin resistance
Body mass index: 25 kg/m^2
Waist circumference: Less than 100 cm

ROLE OF DIET IN DIABETES

A healthy diet plays an important role in preventing and managing diabetes. Preventing diabetes isn't just about avoiding foods that can spike your blood sugar levels, it's also about choosing the right foods that naturally prevent diabetes. In diabetes, moderation and frequency are the keys, you can still eat your favorite foods, but you might need to eat them less often or eat smaller portions.

To prevent and control diabetes:

- Avoid sugary foods that directly raise your blood sugar levels.
- Avoid refined carbohydrates that quickly break down into glucose sugar and raise your blood sugar levels.
- Avoid foods that increase your risk of insulin resistance.
- Avoid foods that increase cholesterol in the body.
- Avoid lifestyle choices that increase the risk of developing diabetes.
- Avoid foods that increase your risk of developing diabetes complications.

Now that you know what type of foods you need to avoid, let's see in the next chapter, which are the top 10 foods and lifestyle choices that you should avoid to prevent and control diabetes.

1.2

10 FOODS THAT INCREASE YOUR DIABETES RISK

Below are the 10 foods that can increase your diabetes risk:

1. Saturated fats

Saturated fats increase the risk of developing type 2 diabetes more than unsaturated fats. Foods that are high in saturated fats, such as butter, cheese, cream, and processed foods like cakes and biscuits can cause high levels of LDL-cholesterol, which increases the risk of cardiovascular diseases in people with diabetes. LDL-cholesterol transports from the liver to the cells, and fat build-up inside muscle cells lowers the insulin response to glucose and increases blood sugar levels, increasing the risk of developing diabetes. Foods like butter, coconut oil, palm oil, and cheese have high amounts of saturated fat.

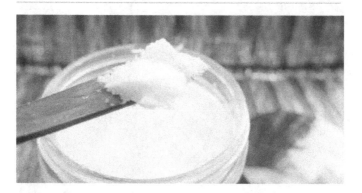

2. Starchy foods

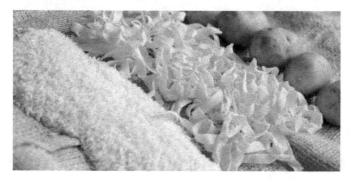

Starchy foods such as white rice, boiled potatoes, and pasta are high in glycemic index. These foods are quickly digested and absorbed, causing a rapid rise in blood sugar levels. The best way to reduce their effect is to replace them with healthier alternatives. These healthy alternatives contain fiber that is low in the glycemic index. You can replace white rice with brown rice, boiled white potatoes with sweet potatoes, and white pasta with whole wheat pasta or durum wheat pasta. Even though these healthy alternatives provide fiber, you should eat them in moderation.

3. Packaged fruit juices

Packaged fruit juices are high in fructose and low in fiber. It gives a sudden spike in blood sugar and is less nutritious than freshly squeezed juices. Unfortunately, even the healthiest packaged fruit juice in the market can increase insulin resistance and increase your risk of developing diabetes. In fact, not only packaged fruit juices, even fresh fruit juices are not healthy in comparison to fresh fruits. Most of the fibers, vitamins, and anti-oxidants are removed while filtering. So, it is best to eat whole fresh fruit instead of fruit juice.

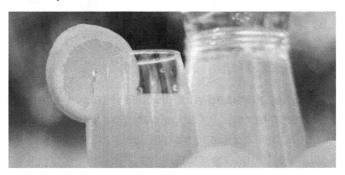

4. Hydrogenated oils

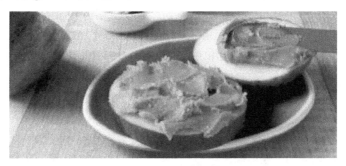

Hydrogenated oils are mainly present in packaged food items such as peanut butter, french fries, margarine, ready-to-use dough, and readymade baked foods. Hydrogenated oils are nothing but healthy vegetable oils that are converted into unhealthier form by the food industry. Vegetable oils are liquids at room temperature, food manufacturers chemically alter the structure of vegetable oils and turn them into solid or spreadable form by adding hydrogen in them. As a result, trans fats are formed. Trans fats increase insulin resistance by affecting cell membrane functions and increase your risk of developing type 2 diabetes. They are a major contributor to heart disease because they are highly inflammatory and can increase your LDL-cholesterol (bad) while lowering your HDL-cholesterol (good).

5. Tobacco use

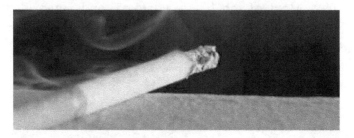

Tobacco use may fluctuate your glucose levels by altering the way your body uses glucose. Tobacco contains an addictive chemical called nicotine that increases insulin resistance, which can lead to type 2 diabetes. Tobacco stimulates the secretion of a steroid hormone called cortisol, which increases the production of glucose by the liver and makes fat and muscle cells resistant to the action of insulin. The more you smoke, the higher your risk of developing diabetes. Smokers have almost double the risk of developing diabetes compared with people who don't smoke.

6. Alcohol

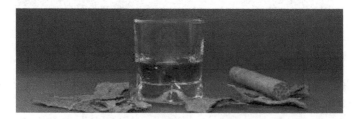

Excess alcohol intake increases your risk of developing type 2 diabetes. Alcohol contains a lot of calories, which can make you obese. Obesity increases insulin resistance, which can lead to diabetes or can worsen your diabetes condition. Another disadvantage of drinking alcohol is that it produces a synergic effect and causes hypoglycemia by interacting with some of your prescribed anti-diabetic medicines such as sulfonylureas. Typically, the liver releases stored glucose when blood sugar levels drop, to maintain normal blood glucose, and to prevent hypoglycemia. But when you drink alcohol, it interferes with the way liver works and reduces the liver's ability to recover the dropped blood glucose levels. It results in hypoglycemia.

7. Soda

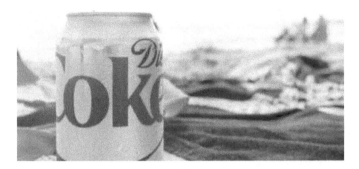

Soda and sugar-sweetened energy drinks can increase your diabetes risk, and if you already have diabetes, you must totally avoid them. The high sugar content of these drinks causes rapid spikes in blood sugar levels. These sugary drinks contain lots of calories, which can make you obese. The excess body weight makes your muscles, liver, and fat cells resistant to the insulin's signals of grabbing glucose out of the bloodstream. The high sugar levels in your blood make your pancreas to release more and more insulin to overcome the body's resistance and to maintain the blood sugar levels normal. Over time, this affects the pancreas's ability to make sufficient insulin, and your blood sugar begins to rise, and you develop diabetes.

8. Full fat dairy

Full-fat milk and milk products can increase the levels of cholesterol in the blood and lead to a higher risk of cardiovascular diseases. High-fat content can also lead to insulin resistance. Avoid eating full-fat milk, butter, full-fat yogurt, full-fat ice cream, and cheese. Even skimmed milk contains carbohydrates and can affect your blood sugar levels, but you should not completely avoid milk because it contains nutrients, which are a must for your body to function properly. It is better to remove other high calories and sugary food sources from your diet than milk.

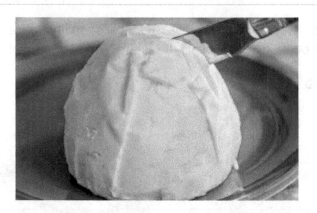

9. Salt

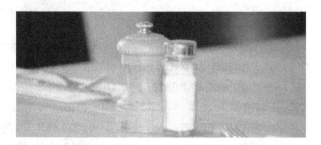

It is crucial to maintain normal blood pressure in diabetes. Salt does not directly affect blood glucose levels, but you should limit your salt consumption for managing diabetes efficiently. Too much salt can raise your blood pressure. High blood pressure with diabetes increases your risk of cardiovascular diseases. You should maintain your blood pressure less than 130/80 mm Hg. You must limit your table salt consumption to 5g or one teaspoon per day to prevent and control diabetes.

10. Certain drugs

Certain drugs such as corticosteroids and pain-relieving non-steroidal anti-inflammatory drugs (NSAIDs) are contradicted in diabetes. Oral Corticosteroids can increase blood glucose levels and cause insulin resistance by reducing the sensitivity of the cells toward insulin. Corticosteroids can worsen diabetes conditions; this is why people with diabetes, as well as individuals with pre-diabetes, should avoid them.

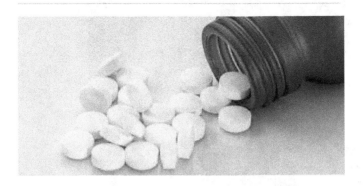

People with diabetes who are receiving sulfonylureas drugs should avoid taking a high dose of pain-relieving non-steroidal anti-inflammatory drugs (NSAIDs) such as ibuprofen. One of the side effects of sulfonylureas is hypoglycemia means it lowers the blood sugar levels than the normal range. NSAIDs affect the ion channel functions of beta cells that secrete insulin. When you take NSAIDs together with sulphonylureas, it induces hypoglycemia.

CONCLUSION

These were the foods and lifestyle choices that you must avoid or at least limit the consumption to prevent diabetes, but as I said before, just avoiding harmful foods is not enough in managing diabetes. You must eat the right nutrition; in fact, eating foods that naturally prevent and even treat your diabetes is more important than just avoiding harmful foods. Diabetes-friendly foods not only can help control blood sugar levels, but some of them can even repair beta cells and can increase your insulin sensitivity. With regular consumption of these foods, your body naturally builds a defense system against diabetes, and you control diabetes without medicines or with a reduced dose of your medications.

Now let's see which are the top 10 best foods that can help you prevent and control diabetes without medicines.

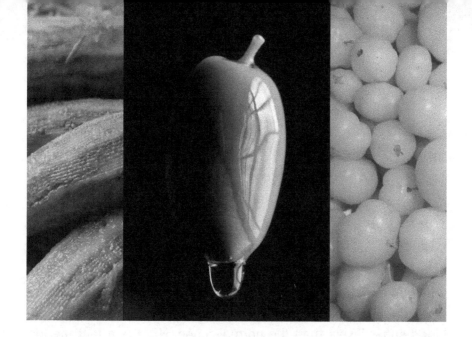

1.3

10 BEST FOODS TO PREVENT AND CONTROL DIABETES

Below are 10 best foods to prevent and control diabetes:

1. Bitter gourd (bitter melon)

Bitter gourd (bitter melon) contains compounds that help lower blood glucose and fats levels in the body. Bitter gourd juice is an excellent beverage for people with diabetes. In fact, it is more effective than some second-line drugs for controlling glucose levels in the body. It works through various mechanisms to lower blood sugar levels. It limits the breakdown of the carbohydrates into glucose by inhibiting the carbohydrates metabolizing enzymes.

Furthermore, bitter gourd enhances the glucose uptake by tissues and increases glucose metabolism. It repairs damaged beta cells that make insulin and prevents their death. It contains chemical compounds such as charantin and polypeptide-p that exhibit a hypoglycemic effect. Polypeptide-p or p-insulin is an insulin-like protein. It works by mimicking the action of insulin in the body and very effective in controlling sugar levels in patients with type-1 diabetes.

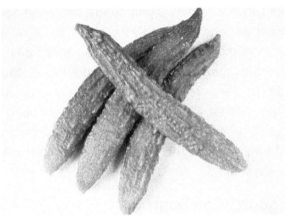

Bitter gourd helps in treating obesity by boosting the system and enzymes responsible for converting fat into energy. It prevents the accumulation of fat in the body, which prevents fat-induced insulin resistance. In season, you must eat at least one medium bitter gourd or 50-100 ml of bitter gourd juice in a day. Bitter gourd could be your magic pill to reduce your dependence on your anti-diabetic medications. If you are healthy and young but have a family history of diabetes, then you should start eating bitter gourd to prevent diabetes in the future.

2. Fenugreek seeds

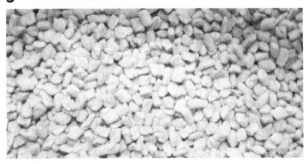

Fenugreek seeds are the second most effective food, after bitter gourd to control diabetes naturally. Regular consumption of fenugreek seeds effectively prevents the development of diabetes. Fenugreek seeds increase glucose-induced insulin release. The research finding shows that after consumption of fenugreek seeds soaked in hot water, significantly decrease fasting blood sugar, triglyceride, and LDL-cholesterol up to 30%. If you have diabetes, you should eat fenugreek seeds every day. But before you start eating them, consult your doctor because regular consumption of fenugreek seed decreases your blood sugar levels, and you need a lesser dose of your prescribed drug. Soak fenugreek seeds in a cup of water overnight. The next morning on an empty stomach, chew the seeds and drink the water in which the seeds were soaked.

3. Bottle gourd/Calabash

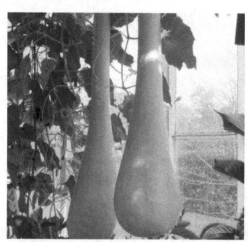

Consumption of bottle gourd helps reduce blood sugar levels. Bottle gourd is very low in calories and high in both soluble and insoluble dietary fiber. It contains almost 90% water, which makes it a choice of vegetable in diabetes. Bottle gourd helps prevent the development of insulin resistance in type 2 diabetes. It inhibits the action of an enzyme called protein-tyrosine phosphatase (PTP) 1B, which improves glucose metabolism and enhances insulin sensitivity without causing lipid accumulation in the liver and thus helps in obesity control.

Make sure you don't eat bitter bottle gourd. First taste a piece of bottle gourd before cooking, discard it if it is bitter because bitter bottle gourd is not edible and can even cause toxicity and stomach ulcer.

4. Barley

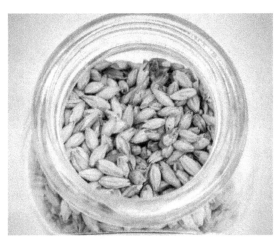

If you want to prevent diabetes, start eating barley regularly. The lower consumption of dietary fiber is associated with the increasing prevalence of diabetes. Barley is an excellent source of soluble fiber along with antioxidant minerals such as magnesium, copper, selenium, and chromium. Research shows long term consumption of barley is effective in lowering blood glucose levels by mimicking the mechanism of action of your first line anti-diabetes drugs. It decreases insulin resistance and interferes with carbohydrates absorption and metabolism. Carbohydrates in barley convert into glucose gradually, without rapidly increasing blood glucose levels. It increases a hormone that helps reduce chronic low-grade inflammation. Barley is an incredible preventive food for those who are at high risk for developing diabetes. You can grind barley and make flour. Add barley flour in wheat flour whenever you make chapati or bread; you can even add barley flour to your cake batter.

5. Monounsaturated fats

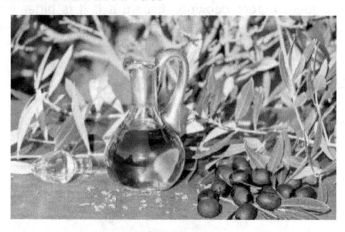

Monounsaturated fats such as olive oil, canola oil, and avocado can be advantageous for those with type 1 or type 2 diabetes who are trying to lose or maintain weight. High-monounsaturated-fat diets cause a modest increase in HDL-cholesterol levels, and lower LDL-cholesterol levels, as well as improve glycemic control. Oil containing monounsaturated fats is the choice of oil in diabetes, so choose your cooking oil accordingly. You can protect your heart by replacing saturated fats in your diet with monounsaturated fats. Regular consumption of monounsaturated fats prevents insulin resistance and accumulation of abdominal fat by increasing your fat-burning hormone adiponectin. Keep in mind that oils are high in calories, even the healthiest oils, so consume them in moderation. Your objective should be to replace saturated fats with monounsaturated fats. Keep the intake of polyunsaturated fats (soybean oil, sunflower oil, and corn oil) less than 10% of total energy consumption. Your total fat consumption should be less than 35% of total energy consumption (from carbohydrates and protein).

6. Legumes

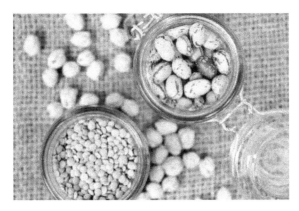

Legumes are a superfood for people with diabetes. Legumes such as chickpeas, kidney beans, and peas help manage and reduce type 2 diabetes risk. They are low on the glycemic index (GI) scale despite containing carbohydrates. They increase serum adiponectin concentrations in type 2 diabetic patients that help in preventing abdominal fat and reduce the risk of insulin resistance. Always choose dried beans over canned beans because lots of salt is added in canned products, which can increase your risk of high blood pressure. If you must use canned beans, be sure to rinse them to get rid of salt as much as possible.

7. Zinc

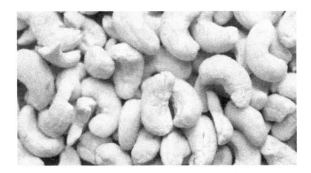

Zinc plays an antioxidant role in type 2 diabetes. It improves oxidative stress by reducing chronic hyperglycemia. It has been seen that people with diabetes have lower levels of zinc than people without diabetes. Zinc deficiency may lead to the development of diabetes. It is because zinc plays a crucial part in insulin metabolism; it helps in the production and secretion of insulin. As zinc strengthens the immune system, it protects beta cells from destruction.

Moreover, zinc prevents diabetes by increasing the levels of adiponectin hormone in the body that helps reduce weight. Studies suggest zinc-rich foods help lower blood sugar levels in type 1 as well as type 2 diabetes. Foods that are high in zinc are cashew nuts, sesame seeds, chickpeas, kidney beans, milk, and oats.

8. Fruits

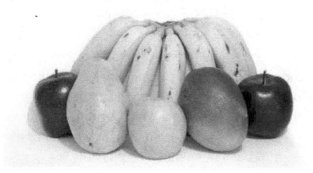

Because of the sugar content, generally, people with diabetes avoid fruits, which is not right. Fruits are full of soluble fiber and don't contain free sugar that is found in chocolate, cakes, biscuits, fruit juices, and cold drinks. So, if you want to cut down the sugar intake, avoid fruit juices, sugary drinks, and cakes than whole fruits. You can easily have one large banana or a medium apple or one slice of papaya in a day.

9. Low-fat yogurt

Probiotics help to reduce inflammation in the body. Yogurt is the best example of probiotics. Yogurt is low in carbohydrates and contains a good amount of protein, vitamin D, calcium, and potassium. It reduces fasting blood glucose, blood pressure, lipid profile, and other cardiovascular risk factors in people with type 2 diabetes.

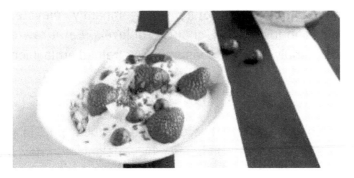

Probiotics control the glycemic condition by lowering insulin resistance and decreasing the production of inflammatory markers. People who eat yogurt have better control over blood sugar in comparison to those who do not eat yogurt. Choose low-fat yogurt over regular yogurt to prevent weight gain.

10. Indian gooseberry/ Amla

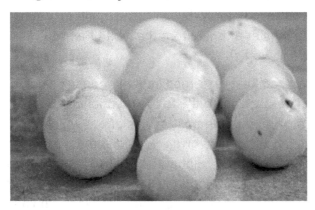

The Indian gooseberry is the richest source of vitamin C, containing 20 times more vitamin C than that of orange. Vitamin C lowers blood pressure in people with type 2 diabetes and protects your heart. Indian gooseberry is rich in nutrients and phytochemicals, such as gallic acid, ellagic acid, gallotannin, and corilagin. These all are potent antioxidants. Through their free radical scavenging properties, these phytochemicals help prevent and control hyperglycemia, cardiac complications, and diabetic complications like nephropathy and neuropathy. Amla favorably impacts on the lipid profile, it significantly elevates HDL-cholesterol and lowers LDL-cholesterol levels. Eat it raw or make chutney or simply boil and consume the strained amla juice.

CONCLUSION

Type 2 diabetes is a lifestyle disease. The best part is you can prevent and control diabetes by making some lifestyle modifications. Lack of awareness and over-promotion of unhealthy foods and bad lifestyle choices are the reason why the incidence of diabetes is increasing in population. There is no harm in enjoying unhealthy foods, considering you are consuming them in moderation. Whether or not your blood sugar level is high, to effectively prevent diabetes, reduce your frequency of eating out. Eat homemade foods. Make every unhealthy food at home, and make it from scratch. By the end, when your food will be ready to eat, you will involuntarily fill with the guilt of eating so many unhealthy things at a time. From the next time, you will crave less. Try this trick, it works!

If you are on diabetes medications, consult your doctor and pharmacist before adding the foods mentioned above in your diet. They can provide you the best advice about which foods you can eat and which ones not, given your diabetes condition and the complications of your diabetes. When you eat the foods mentioned above, your blood glucose levels drop, and you need a lesser dose of medicines. So, regularly discuss with your doctor to adjust the dose accordingly, sometimes doctors just repeat the previous prescription in a hurry without checking your current blood sugar levels.

KEY POINTS

✓ Regularly check your blood pressure. Maintain blood pressure <130/80 mm Hg. Tight control of blood pressure can be more effective than glycemic control in preventing heart disease.

✓ Be active. Play outdoor games, use stairs, don't sit for long. A sedentary lifestyle leads to obesity, which causes insulin resistance.

✓ Increase adiponectin (fat burning hormone) levels in your body by eating monounsaturated fats.

✓ Don't just add additional monounsaturated fats in your diet, instead replace saturated fats with monounsaturated fats.

✓ Drink plenty of water. Water helps remove excess sugar from your blood through urine.

✓ Eat foods that contain soluble fiber and complex carbohydrates that are low in the glycemic index. You can typically eat protein, but proteins are restricted in people who have or are at risk of kidney damage.

✓ Keep an eye on your hypoglycemia symptoms. Always keep some glucose tablets with you.

✓ If you have diabetes, avoid diabetes complications by getting regular diabetes tests, which can catch problems early and can help you prevent serious diabetes complications. Get a yearly eye exam to ensure no blood vessels of the retina has damaged. Get your cholesterol levels checked. Get a regular urine microalbumin tests to check your kidneys' health, and, electrocardiogram to check your heart health.

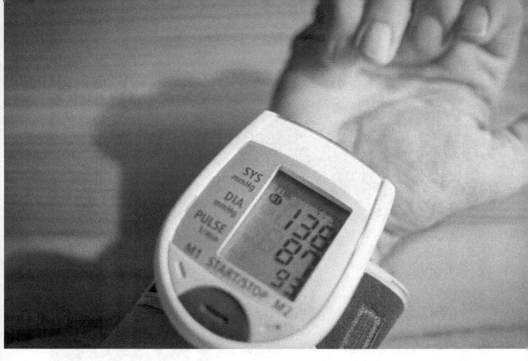

2

HYPERTENSION

2.1

EVERYTHING YOU NEED TO KNOW ABOUT HYPERTENSION

Hypertension is also known as high blood pressure, is a medical condition that can increase your risk of heart disease, stroke, and other severe health complications. The heart pumps blood into arteries (blood vessels) that carry blood away from the heart to the tissues and organs of the body. Blood pressure is the measure of the force of blood against blood vessel walls. When the force of the blood against the artery walls is too high, it increases the blood pressure, and this condition is known as hypertension.

It is dangerous and needs to be controlled because high blood pressure makes the heart work harder to pump blood out to the organs. This can result in hardening of the arteries (atherosclerosis), stroke, kidney disease, and heart failure.

Blood pressure is expressed by two measurements, maximum and minimum pressures, or a top number and bottom number. Let's see what these numbers are:

Systolic blood pressure - Top number (maximum pressure) tells your systolic pressure. When the heartbeats, it contracts and pumps blood through the arteries to the rest of the body, the contraction creates pressure on blood vessels. This is called systolic blood pressure. Normal systolic pressure is below 120 millimeters of mercury (mm Hg). A reading of 130 mm Hg or higher means high blood pressure.

Diastolic blood pressure - Bottom number (minimum pressure) tells your diastolic pressure. The heart contracts to pump blood to the rest of the body and relaxes before it contracts again. The resting time between beats is when your heart fills with blood and gets oxygen. Diastolic pressure is the pressure of the blood in the arteries when the heart is filling. Normal diastolic pressure is below 80 millimeters of mercury (mm Hg). A reading of 80 mm Hg or higher means high blood pressure.

Among both the numbers, systolic blood pressure is more important than diastolic blood pressure because systolic blood pressure gives the best idea of your risk of having a heart attack or a stroke.

CLASSIFICATION OF BLOOD PRESSURE

Classification of blood pressure for adults aged 18 and older as per ACC/AHA (American College of Cardiology and American Heart Association) and ESC/ESH (European Society of Cardiology and the European Society of Hypertension).

As per ACC/AHA			As per ESC/ESH		
Category	Systolic (mmHg)	Diastolic (mmHg)	Category	Systolic (mmHg)	Diastolic (mmHg)
Normal	Less than 120	Less than 80	Optimal	Less than 120	Less than 80
Elevated	120-129	Less than 80	Normal	120-129	80-84
			High normal	130-139	85-89
Hypertension stage 1	130-139	80-89	Hypertension Grade 1	140-159	90-99
Hypertension stage 2	Equal or more than 140	Equal or more than 90	Hypertension Grade 2	160-179	100-109
			Hypertension Grade 3	Equal or more than 180	Equal or more than 110

As per **ESC/ESH** blood pressure level, **140/90 mm Hg** count as hypertension, whereas new guidelines of **ACC/AHA** count **130/80** mm Hg as hypertension. It is because of a new study that has found that blood pressure levels between 130/80 mm Hg to 139/89 mm Hg is enough to cause substantial heart and blood vessel complications.

SYMPTOMS OF HIGH BLOOD PRESSURE

In high blood pressure, it is quite possible that you won't experience any symptoms for years or even decades, this is the reason why hypertension count as a silent killer. However, once blood pressure reaches in hypertension stage, a person may have the following symptoms:

- Severe headache (specifically on the back of the head in the morning)
- Chest pain
- Shortness of breath
- Fatigue and confusion
- Vision problems
- Blood in the urine
- Flushing
- Pounding in your chest or neck

The best way to determine whether your blood pressure is high or not is to voluntarily ask your doctor to check your BP when you go for a health check-up. You should get your BP checked every four months. If your blood pressure is elevated, do get checked every month. If you have high blood pressure and you are on medicines, you should check your BP twice a day. The first measurement should be in the morning before eating or taking any medications, and the second in the evening. Each time you measure, take two or three readings at an interval of 1 or 2 mins to make sure your results are accurate.

Let's first understand what actually happens in the body that causes blood pressure to rise.

MECHANISMS THROUGH WHICH BLOOD PRESSURE RISES

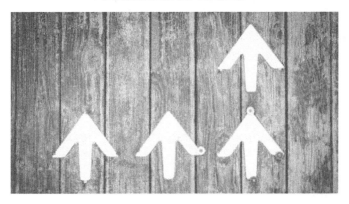

1. Abnormalities of the sympathetic nervous system

You must have heard it many times "*do not stress, or else your blood pressure will go up,*" and it's absolutely right." The sympathetic nervous system influences the blood vessels of the body in a dangerous or stressful condition. When you stress out, sympathetic outflow increases. The sympathetic nervous system release the hormones adrenaline and noradrenaline (also known as norepinephrine). These hormones increase the rate of blood pumping from the heart to deliver fresh oxygen to the brain and muscles. The repeated stress means a continuous increase in blood pumping from the heart, which is attained by constricting the blood vessels. The constant constriction of the blood vessels causes the narrowing of the blood vessels and increases the resistance of the blood vessels to blood flow (peripheral resistance). As a result, blood pressure increases.

2. Abnormalities in the intrarenal renin-angiotensin-aldosterone system (RAAS)

This system controls blood pressure by regulating the volume of fluids in the body. When blood flow to the kidneys decreases, the kidneys secrete enzyme renin into blood circulation. Plasma renin then converts angiotensinogen to angiotensin I, which have no direct biological activity. However, an enzyme known as Angiotensin-Converting Enzyme (ACE) converts Angiotensin I to Angiotensin II (the primary hormone responsible for high blood pressure). Angiotensin II is a peptide hormone that causes vasoconstriction, which means it contracts the muscular wall of the vessels, which causes the narrowing of the blood vessels, resulting in increased blood pressure.

RISK FACTORS

Below are the contributory factors that increase your blood pressure:
- Stress
- Obesity
- Excess alcohol
- Smoking
- Family history of high blood pressure
- Excess salt intake
- A diet lack of potassium
- Lack of exercise
- Certain drugs such as NSAIDs, steroids and contraceptive pills

WHY IS HYPERTENSION DANGEROUS?

Hypertension or High Blood Pressure is dangerous because it causes other health complications. Blood vessels are responsible for delivering oxygen and nutrients to vital organs and tissues. Over time, high blood pressure damages the blood vessels. The damaged blood vessels disrupt the blood flow in the body that cause other health problems to arise. The most affected part of the body by hypertension is heart, followed by, brain, kidney, and reproductive system.

Damage to the arteries
Blood vessels that carry oxygen-rich blood from the heart to the body are called arteries. Arteries are flexible, elastic, and their inner lining is smooth. Blood flows freely and unobstructed through healthy arteries and supply oxygen and nutrients to vital organs and tissues. High blood pressure reduces the elasticity of arteries. It damages their inner lining that makes it easier for dietary fats to collect in the damaged arteries, limiting blood flow throughout your body. These blockages eventually can lead to heart attack and stroke.

Damage to the heart
Hypertension makes your heart pump more frequently, and with more force than a healthy heart, which causes part of your heart (left ventricle) to thicken. An enlarged heart increases your risk of heart attack, heart failure, and sudden cardiac death.

Also, high blood pressure damages the vessels that supply blood to your heart. When blood flow to your heart is obstructed, it can cause arrhythmia (irregular heart rhythms), angina (chest pain), or can cause a heart attack.

Damage to the brain
Our brain depends on nourishing oxygen-rich blood supply to work properly. But high blood pressure can reduce blood and oxygen supply to the brain that can cause several problems, including:

Transient ischemic attack (TIA): Hardened arteries or blood clots caused by high blood pressure can temporarily disrupt the blood supply to the brain, which is called a transient ischemic attack (TIA) or mini-stroke. TIA count as a warning of a full-blown stroke.

Stroke: High blood pressure can cause blood clots to form in the arteries, leading to significant blockages in blood flow. Reduced blood flow makes the brain deprived of oxygen and nutrients, causing brain cells to die. This is known as a stroke.

Dementia: Certain types of dementia, such as vascular dementia, is caused by a lack of blood flow in the brain, which may have caused by narrowed/blocked arteries or due to a stroke.

Damage to the kidneys

Kidneys filter excess fluid and waste from the blood. High blood pressure damages the blood vessels in and leading to your kidneys. Damaged vessels obstruct the blood flow to the kidneys and prevent kidneys from effectively filtering waste from your blood, allowing dangerous waste to accumulate. Hypertension is one of the most common causes of kidney failure.

Damage to the eyes

High blood pressure can damage the blood vessels that supply blood to your eyes. Limited blood flow can damage the retina and the optic nerve, leading to bleeding in the eye, blurred vision, and even complete loss of vision.

MECHANISM THROUGH WHICH ANTI-HYPERTENSIVE MEDICINES WORK

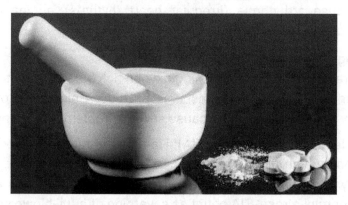

The primary purpose of all the anti-hypertensive drugs is to produce vasodilation means to make the blood vessels wider or more open. When blood vessels dilate, blood freely flows through them, causing a fall in blood pressure.

There are different mechanisms through which different classes of drugs achieve vasodilation. Let's see in brief how do these drugs work and how can we produce similar effect through foods, which are safer and have no side effects:

The first-line therapy or most common drugs that are used in hypertension lower the blood pressure by decreasing the salt reabsorption in the kidneys. That means your body now has less salt because more and more salt, along with water, are flushed out from the body through urine. Because you have less fluid in your blood vessels, the pressure inside will be lower. The drugs that work on this mechanism are called Diuretics. Our aim is to include foods that naturally have a diuretic effect. We will later see in detail about the foods that are natural diuretics.

As we discussed above, the Angiotensin II hormone is the main culprit behind high blood pressure. So, the other class of drugs produces vasodilation either by blocking the conversion of angiotensin I to angiotensin II (ACE inhibitors drugs) or by blocking the actions of angiotensin II (Angiotensin receptor blockers drugs). This allows blood vessels to widen and relax, making it easier for blood to flow through, which lowers your blood pressure.

Calcium stimulates the heart to contract more forcefully. A class of drugs called calcium channel blockers limits the rate at which calcium flows into the cells of the heart and blood vessel walls. As a result, blood vessels widen, and your heart doesn't have to work as hard to pump, making it easier for blood to flow through, and your blood pressure lowers.

STRATEGY TO PREVENT AND CONTROL HYPERTENSION

Hypertension is food and lifestyle-related disease that means foods play the most significant part in correcting as well as worsening the condition. Hypertension cannot be solely managed with medicines. Certain diet and lifestyle modifications are must for controlling the disease effectively. Medications prescribed in hypertension have side effects that include erectile impotence, gout, cough, and lack of energy. By adding the right foods for high blood pressure in your diet and avoiding the bad foods, you can effectively lower your blood pressure and can drastically reduce the dose of your blood pressure medicines.

Below are certain ways by which you can lower your blood pressure naturally:

- Eat foods that reduce sodium levels in the body.
- Exclude foods that silently add salt in your body.
- Eat foods that are naturally diuretic.
- Eat foods that reduce fluid retention in the body and increase urine production.
- Eat foods that are rich in magnesium as magnesium is a natural calcium channel blocker.
- Eat foods that are rich in potassium because potassium negates the sodium effect.
- Eat foods rich in nitrates, which convert into nitric oxide in your body. Nitric oxide widens the blood vessels and lowers blood pressure.
- By increasing water intake.

SALT

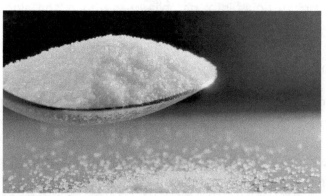

It must have come to your mind that why is it said to avoid table salt in hypertension? What is the exact relationship between salt and blood pressure? So, let's see why salt is dangerous for blood pressure.

Sodium is the main reason for rising blood pressure, and your table salt is basically a combination of sodium (40%) and chloride (60%). Are salt and sodium the same? No, not exactly. Sodium is a mineral that occurs naturally in foods. With table salt, you eat sodium in the form of sodium chloride. This is the reason why table salt considered dangerous for high blood pressure.

Other forms of sodium that you consume are
- Sodium bicarbonate (baking soda) and
- Monosodium glutamate (MSG): Generally used as salt in Chinese foods.

HOW DOES SALT INCREASE BLOOD PRESSURE?

Eating salt raises the amount of sodium in your bloodstream. It affects the performance of your kidneys to remove the water. As a result, your body holds extra water to flush out the extra sodium from your body. This is called fluid retention. The excess fluid in the body puts stress on blood vessels and heart and causes blood pressure to rise.

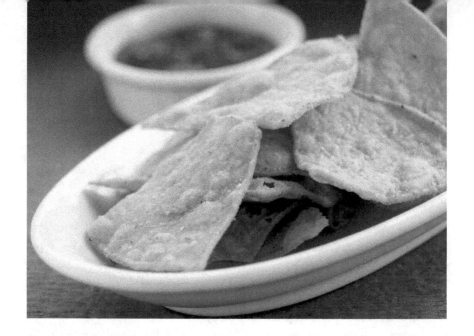

2.2

10 FOODS THAT RAISE YOUR BLOOD PRESSURE

Foods that are high in calories increase cholesterol in your body, which raises blood pressure. Some foods silently add salt to your body and increase your risk of high blood pressure. You don't even release that you are eating salt. To help you identify these foods, here's a list of 10 foods and drinks that knowingly or silently add salt and cholesterol in your body and can raise your blood pressure.

1. Canned foods or beverages

Canned food products are prepared with lots of salt to preserve the food from decaying, and for taste. This decreases the nutrition of the food and silently add salt in your body. For example, as such, chickpeas are very nutritious and have great health benefits, but if you are using canned chickpeas, then they are harmful to your health. Whenever possible, eat fresh foods instead of canned ones. Even if you are using canned chickpeas or other canned vegetables, wash them properly before use to remove the extra salt. Cans are often lined with the chemical bisphenol A (BPA). Eating foods from cans lined with the chemical bisphenol A (BPA) could raise your blood pressure.

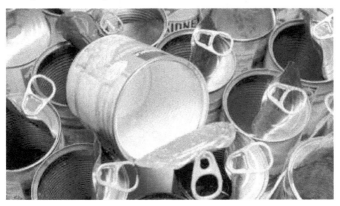

2. Deep-fried foods

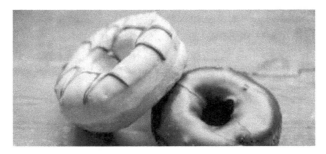

Eating deep-fried foods, such as french fries, bagels, and puris, increases your risk of high blood pressure, heart attack, and stroke. Fried foods add a lot of calories and deficient in healthy nutrients. These increase cholesterol levels in the body and raise your blood pressure. You should never reuse the oil that has been used in deep frying, also don't fry at high temperature. When you deep fry, oils break down with each frying, and their composition changes. As a result, a chemical is formed in food that can lead to cancer.

3. Pickles

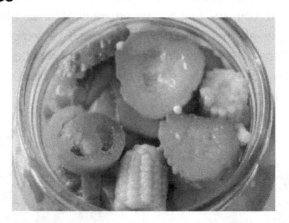

Eating pickles can raise your blood pressure. Lots of salt and oil are required for preserving pickles for long. Salt and oil stop the food from decaying and keep them edible for long. Adding extra sodium of pickle to your diet causes water retention that puts greater pressure on blood vessels and increases blood pressure. Furthermore, pickles are loaded with excess oil that can increase cholesterol in your body. Cholesterol can narrow the blood vessels that prevent the free-flowing of blood and make it harder for the heart to pump blood through them. As a result, your blood pressure rises.

4. Processed cheese

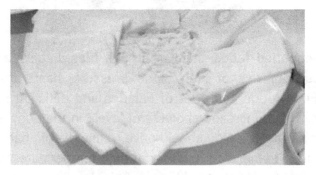

Processed cheese is high on calories and salt. This means regular consumption can lead to high cholesterol, obesity, and high blood pressure, increasing your risk of heart disease. Avoid eating too much-processed cheese. Instead of processed cheese, go for homemade cottage cheese. You can even eat mozzarella cheese as it contains the lowest salt in comparison to other varieties. Cheese can offer health benefits as they are rich in calcium and vitamins. However, if you have diagnosed with high blood pressure, avoid eating any cheese except homemade low-fat cottage cheese (not the store-bought).

5. Caffeine

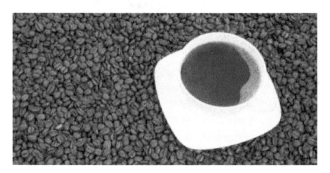

Your one cup of coffee may give a boost to start your day in an active mode, but it is not good for blood pressure. Caffeine increases the release of the hormone adrenaline, which is responsible for making you active within some minutes of consumption. However, this same hormone adrenaline causes constriction of blood vessels and increases the rate and force of heart pumping. As a result, pressure inside your blood vessels increases. Don't quit tea or coffee completely, instead gradually reduce the frequency, and soon your body will adapt it. Quitting the caffeine all of a sudden will only make you more crave for it.

6. Dehydration

Keep yourself hydrated. When your body is dehydrated, your brain sends a signal to the pituitary gland to secrete hormone vasopressin, which is an antidiuretic hormone. It constricts the blood vessels. As a result, pressure inside the blood vessels increases, which leads to hypertension. Drink at least eight glasses of water in a day. Drinking enough water in pregnancy is essential, especially if your blood pressure is already high, to prevent toxemia, which is a potentially dangerous pregnancy complication characterized by the onset of high blood pressure.

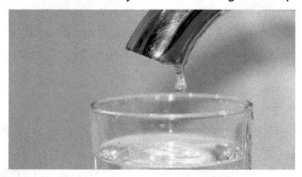

7. Smoking

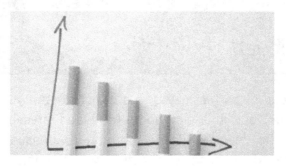

Each cigarette you smoke increases your blood pressure. The nicotine in cigarettes is the main reason for high blood pressure. Nicotine stimulates the central nervous system. High blood pressure is caused by both an increase in cardiac output and total peripheral vascular resistance. Nicotine acts as a stimulant in the body. It stimulates the adrenal glands to release more adrenaline. It forces the heart to constrict more forcefully, which affects the heart pumping capacity. It narrows your blood vessels and hardens their walls. As a result, your blood flow gets restricted, which increases peripheral vascular resistance and makes your blood more likely to clot. If you smoke, quit it as soon as possible—people who quit smoking live longer than people who smoke.

8. Alcohol

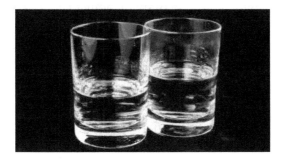

Any alcoholic beverage can increase your blood pressure. Alcohol interferes with the effectiveness of your anti-hypertensive drugs. In fact, even one drink can change the way your blood pressure medications work and increase the side effects of blood pressure medications.

Alcohol increases blood pressure by increasing cortisol (stress hormone) levels. Alcohol stimulates the release of vasoconstrictor angiotensin II and induces inflammation that inhibits nitric oxide production in the body. Alcohol is high in calories and may contribute to unwanted weight gain, which is a risk factor for high blood pressure. If you want to prevent high blood pressure, quit drinking completely.

9. Sugar

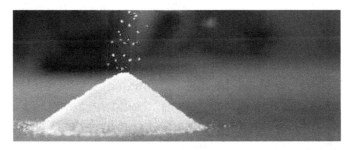

It might surprise you, but high sugar intake is linked with hypertension. Not only because it leads to obesity, but it causes high blood pressure through a different mechanism too. Sugar elevates uric acid in the body that induces oxidative stress and decreases endothelial nitric oxide availability. It also activates both renin activity and angiotensin activity in the kidney. Nitric oxide suppression, as well as enhancement of angiotensin activity, constricts the blood vessels, leading to high blood pressure. Sugar also gives empty calories and increases cholesterol in the body. Increased cholesterol causes plaque to build up inside your arteries, and arteries become hardened and narrowed. As a result, your heart has to work much harder to pump blood through them and cause an increase in your blood pressure.

10. Packaged snacks

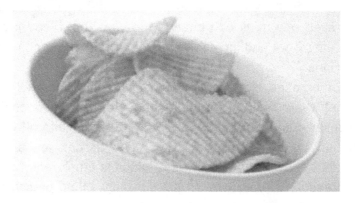

Potato chips, popcorns, sev, banana chips, and other packaged snacks have lots of salt in it. More the flavors, the more the salt content. Flavors like salted, cream, and onion have more salt content. Additionally, these are high in saturated and trans fats, sugar, and other low-fiber carbohydrates. Consuming too much of packaged snacks increases bad cholesterol (LDL) in the body. High LDL levels may lead to the formation of cholesterol plaque in the blood vessel that constricts the free-flowing of blood and may eventually lead to the development of coronary heart disease. You don't need to stop eating snacks completely, but do limit your servings and frequency. Look for plain version instead of flavored.

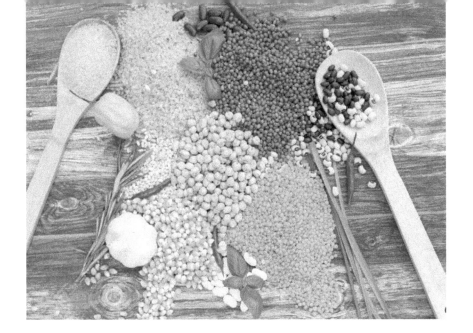

2.3

10 FOODS THAT LOWER BLOOD PRESSURE JUST LIKE ANTIHYPERTENSIVE DRUGS

Certain foods naturally lower blood pressure. Adding these foods in your diet can significantly reduce your risk of high blood pressure. A diet low in sodium and rich in potassium, magnesium, nitrate, and fiber can help prevent and control blood pressure.

Below are the top 10 foods that work just like antihypertensive drugs and lower your blood pressure:

1. Leafy green vegetables

Leafy green vegetables such as spinach, kale, fennel, and cabbage are very dense in nutrition. These are packed with potassium, magnesium, nitrates, and full of fiber. Low potassium intake is one of the risk factors in developing high blood pressure. The potassium content of leafy green vegetables flushes out sodium. The rich magnesium content act as calcium channel antagonist, modulating vascular tone and reactivity that dilates blood vessels. As a result, blood flows without any restriction through your blood vessels, and your blood pressure decreases.

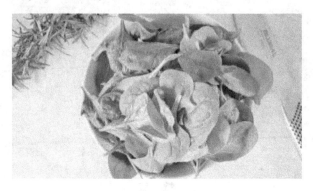

Moreover, nitrate of leafy greens induces vasodilation. Nitrate converts into nitrite in your mouth by oral commensal bacteria. It then converts in nitric oxide in your blood, which relaxes the smooth muscle of your blood vessels and dilates them that allows free-flowing of blood. Prevent using antibacterial mouthwash as it inhibits nitrate to nitrite conversion, and you don't get the blood pressure-lowering benefit of nitric oxide.

2. Beetroot

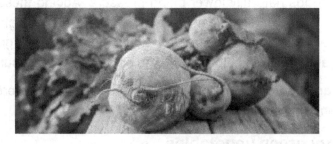

Beetroot is a well-known potent vasodilator. It contains high levels of dietary nitrate; the body converts the nitrate in this vegetable into nitric oxide. Nitric oxide relaxes and dilates blood vessels, so lowering blood pressure. For the full benefit, drink a glass of raw beetroot juice because raw beetroot has more potency than cooked one. Research indicates that within hours of drinking raw beetroot juice, it lowers systolic blood pressure.

3. Garlic

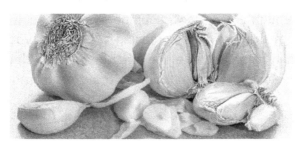

Eating garlic every day may help reduce your blood pressure. The organosulfur compounds of garlic promote vasodilation and lower blood pressure. Garlic lowers blood pressure through various mechanisms of action. Dietary intake of garlic boosts hydrogen sulfide production and regulation of endothelial nitric oxide, which induces smooth muscle cell relaxation and vasodilation; as a result, blood pressure drops. Garlic also blocks angiotensin-II production by inhibition of the angiotensin-converting-enzyme (ACE).

Allicin is an organosulfur compound that releases when garlic is crushed or chopped. Allicin is highly unstable. Cooking speeds up the degradation of allicin, and microwaving destroys it completely.

Eat one clove of freshly crushed garlic empty stomach every day, and it will lower your blood pressure naturally. But keep in mind that raw garlic is quite pungent and can cause burn, so don't hold it in your mouth for long periods. Too much garlic may cause irritation and digestive upset. If you see the irritation, limit the frequency to 2 to 3 times a week.

4. Cucumber

Cucumber is rich in potassium, which plays an important role in regulating blood pressure. The excess sodium in your body reduces the ability of your kidneys to remove the water. This makes your body hold fluids that raises your blood pressure. Potassium lowers blood pressure by balancing out the adverse effects of sodium. The more potassium you eat, the more sodium you lose through urine. Also, cucumber is a diuretic. It flushes out sodium from the body by increasing your urine production and maintain fluid balance in the body that helps keep blood pressure in check. Use cucumber in salad, raita, or have cucumber juice.

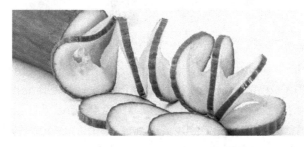

**Read "Secret of Healthy Hair" for a permanent solution to your hair problems.

5. Banana

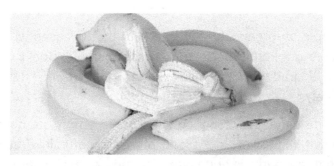

What can be a better source of potassium than the well-known and probably most blood pressure friendly fruit banana! Eating potassium-rich foods decrease sodium levels in your body. It reduces fluid retention and blood pressure by increasing urine production. Potassium also acts as a vasodilator that helps ease tension in your blood vessel walls, which helps lower blood pressure. Banana is one of the healthiest fruits because it is very low in calories and has higher water content.

6. Lemon water

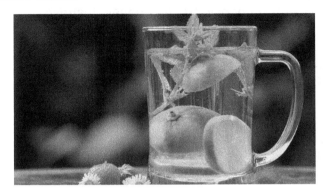

Lemon is an excellent remedy for hypertension as it helps keep blood vessels soft and pliable, making them flexible by removing any rigidity. This keeps the blood pressure low. Lemon is rich in vitamin C that works as an antioxidant and has a diuretic effect. It removes excess fluid from your body, which lowers the blood pressure. Furthermore, vitamin C helps protect the levels of nitric oxide in the body that relaxes blood vessels and contributes to maintaining normal and healthy blood pressure. Taking a glass of warm lemon water every morning on an empty stomach helps you keep the high blood pressure at bay. If you are on blood pressure medicines, do consult your doctor and pharmacist before including citrus fruits like lemon in your diet as citrus fruits can interact with your medications, especially calcium antagonist drugs.

7. Honey

Honey contains antioxidant compounds that are linked to lower blood pressure. Obesity and unhealthy lifestyle cause oxidative stress in your body that reduces vasodilatory agent nitric oxide available in the body. The antioxidants present in honey help to keep the nitric oxide levels high in the body by reducing oxidative stress in the body. Nitric oxide relaxes your blood vessels causing vasodilation, which helps to lower the blood pressure. Take one tablespoon of honey daily or add it in your morning lemon water.

Make sure you eat organic honey, not the processed ones. Eat it raw, don't heat the honey. Heating honey destroys the beneficial enzymes, vitamins, and minerals of the honey.

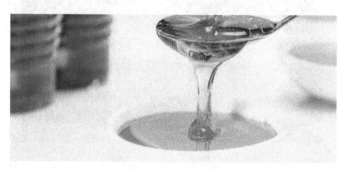

8. Nuts

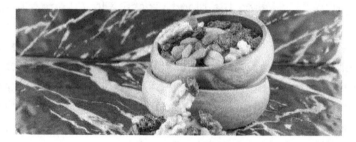

Nuts such as almonds, cashew nuts, and walnuts are rich in magnesium, fiber, and protein. Magnesium is an electrolyte that helps lower high blood pressure. Magnesium is a natural calcium channel blocker, it stimulates the production of vasodilators nitric oxide and prostacyclins. These vasodilators relax the blood vessels and lower blood pressure. Nuts also contain heart-healthy fats that lower cholesterol levels. Remember to get magnesium from your food, not from supplements, to avoid any risk of overdose. Make sure to eat nuts every day.

9. Fenugreek seeds

Drinking fenugreek water can be one of the most effective ways for you to maintain healthy blood pressure. Fenugreek leaves and seeds contain a high amount of dietary fiber. A diet rich in fiber has been linked to steady levels of blood pressure. Dietary fiber is tough to digest. It forms a viscous gel in the intestine that makes it harder for sugars and fats to absorb in the bloodstream and decreases cholesterol levels in the body and prevent weight gain. Furthermore, fenugreek leaves and seeds contain low levels of sodium, which makes it an ideal food for people with high blood pressure.

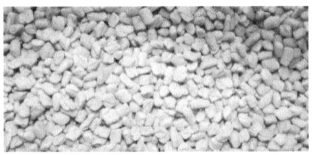

Take two teaspoons of fenugreek seeds and soak them in a glass of water overnight. The next morning remove the seeds from water, drink the fenugreek water on an empty stomach. Crush the seeds to a fine paste and use it in cooking. Do this for at least two to three months and see the positive result yourself.

10. legumes

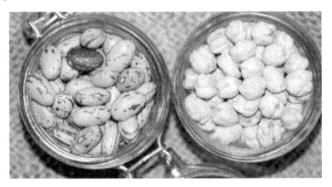

Legumes such as lentils, chickpeas, kidney beans, soybeans, and others, are rich in potassium, magnesium, and fiber. These nutrients maintain healthy and normal blood pressure. Potassium and magnesium in legumes prevent fluid retention, decrease sodium levels by increasing urine production. The soluble fiber in the legumes gets attached to cholesterol particles and takes them out of the body that helps to reduce overall cholesterol levels. This reduces the risk of weight gain and improves vascular health.

IMPLEMENTATION

Now that you know everything about hypertension, how blood pressure works, what exactly goes wrong in your body in hypertension condition, what are the risk factors, what you should avoid and what you should start adding in your diet? Now the question arises, how to implement it?

If you are a healthy person and have no hypertension condition and no family history of hypertension, start with adding foods in your diet that can help you prevent hypertension in the future. Start with adding above mentioned foods that are most of your likening, gradually add those foods in your diet that you do not like much but make sure to add them, gradually you will be habitual. You must add sweet potato, onion, and pomegranate too in your diet; these foods are also very effective in preventing high blood pressure. Limit your consumption of food that increases your risk of high blood pressure. If you smoke, quit it. Limit your alcohol consumption.

If you are a healthy person but have a family history of hypertension, strictly avoid eating known and silent salt-rich foods. With a family history of hypertension, you are susceptible to high blood pressure. Quit smoking and drinking any alcoholic beverages completely, don't increase your risk of high blood pressure. Eat foods as mentioned above that naturally prevent hypertension, also include sweet potato, pomegranate in your diet, but if you have a family history of diabetes too, then limit your consumption of sugar as well as sweet fruits.

If you are a person with high blood pressure, you must eat potassium-rich foods. The best way is to note down all the above mentioned preventive foods, ask your doctor and pharmacist:

I want to add these foods in my diet, is it safe to add all of them? Are there any foods that can interact with my medications? They will provide you the best advice considering your blood pressure levels and other health complications. Let them know if you have other health problems like diabetes and arthritis. If you have diabetes, then limit the consumption of high glycemic foods. If you have arthritis, limit your citrus fruit consumption. After including these foods for three months, ask your doctor, has my blood pressure improved? Do I need the same dose of medicines or lower dose will work? Keep in mind once you have controlled your blood pressure, continue to consume foods that prevent high blood pressure. It should be a lifetime habit, not short-term therapy.

KEY POINTS

✓ Consume less salt. It promotes fluid retention that increases blood pressure.

✓ Avoid foods that silently add salt in your body.

✓ Eat foods low in fat and calories.

✓ Do yoga.

✓ Be active. Physical activity reduces water retention by making you sweat and increasing blood flow to the tissues.

✓ Drink plenty of water, especially on the day you consume more salt. Dehydration can increase your risk of water retention.

✓ Don't stress out.

✓ Eat whole grains instead of refined ones.

✓ Add barley flour to your whole wheat flour in a ratio of 2:10. Add 200 gm of barley flour to 1 kg of whole wheat flour.

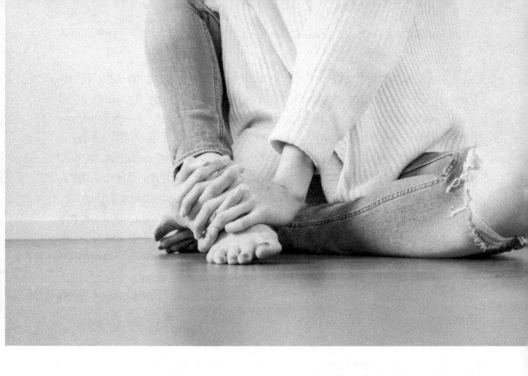

3

<u>ARTHRITIS</u>

3.1

EVERYTHING YOU NEED TO KNOW ABOUT ARTHRITIS

To prevent any disease, first, you need to understand that disease, how that particular disease affects your body, how your body is reacting to disease. What are the points to be taken into consideration while managing that disease? In managing any disease, food and lifestyle play an extremely important role. In a disease condition, the damage that has already been done to the body is out of our control. But limiting the disease's spread and reversing its effect is totally on our hands.

So, let's see how to prevent and manage arthritis.

What is arthritis?

It is a joint disorder featuring inflammation with stiffness and joint pain. It can be of one or more joints—a joint means where two different bones meet for the purpose of permitting body parts to move.

Types of Arthritis

There are more than 100 types of arthritis. Two of the most common types are

Osteoarthritis (OA)

Rheumatoid arthritis (RA)

OSTEOARTHRITIS (OA)

The breakdown of cartilage is called Osteoarthritis. Cartilage is the protective hard, slippery tissue that caps the ends of bones where two bones form a joint. Cartilage cushions the ends of the bones and responsible for smooth and frictionless movement. When this protective layer gets damaged, it results in friction between the bones. The continuous friction causes pain and restricts the joint movement. It mainly occurs in the hands, neck, knees, hips, or lower back.

Causes of Osteoarthritis

Injury to joints or ligaments
- Joint infection
- Diabetes
- Obesity
- Low levels of estrogen hormone in women (mainly after menopause)

RHEUMATOID ARTHRITIS (RA)

Rheumatoid arthritis (RA) is a chronic autoimmune disease in which the immune system mistakenly attacks the joints — mainly the lining of joints (called synovium). This results in inflammation of the affected tissues in and around joints. Eventually, inflammation destroys the joint, and joint loses its shape and alignment.

Rheumatoid arthritis symptoms include:

- Joint pain
- Swollen joints
- Joint stiffness, usually in the mornings
- Fatigue
- Fever
- Joint redness
- Joint deformities

Who is prone to rheumatoid arthritis?

Adults over 55 years
Mostly women
Obese people

What do antirheumatic medications do?

RA medications actually don't treat arthritis but slow the damage that arthritis can cause to your body by

Reducing the pain and
Decreasing the inflammation

The pain-relieving nonsteroidal anti-inflammatory drugs (NSAIDs) reduce pain and inflammation by blocking an enzyme called, COX-2 enzyme and reduce the production of prostaglandins. Prostaglandins are chemicals that promote pain, inflammation, swelling, and fever.

While another class of drugs, disease-modifying antirheumatic drugs (DMARDs) slow down the progression of rheumatoid arthritis by reducing the response of the immune system.

The problem with these drugs is that they may have serious side effects. The RA condition can be easily managed with food therapy. Our motive is to include foods in our diet that are natural COX-2 inhibitors and to exclude foods that promote inflammation in the body.

PREVENTION AND CONTROL OF ARTHRITIS THROUGH FOOD

Diet has a massive impact on arthritis conditions. Some foods cause inflammation in the body, either by increasing free radicals in the body or by enhancing the release of pro-inflammatory proteins. You can prevent arthritis by avoiding any food that causes inflammation in the body. But, for that, you must know the types of foods that cause inflammation or aggravate the pain. Similarly, some foods are potent anti-oxidant and anti-inflammatory. These foods are considered as superfoods for arthritis because they act as natural COX-2 inhibitors and prevent inflammation in the body as well as promote the secretion of the anti-inflammatory protein, which reduce inflammation by preventing oxidative stress in the body.

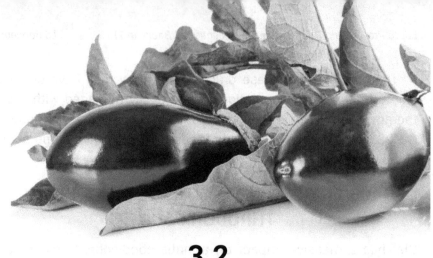

3.2

10 FOODS THAT INCREASE YOUR RISK OF ARTHRITIS OR MAY FLARE UP YOUR ARTHRITIS

Any sour food can flare up your arthritis. Many people have complained that certain foods induce arthritis pain. It can differ from person to person. Some people may experience pain, while others have no effects with these foods. You can check it by yourself, how's your body reacting to these foods. If you experience pain with the following foods, then stop taking them one by one for about 1-2 weeks. If the pain and stiffness go away, that means that particular food is flaring up your arthritis. Don't completely stop taking these foods but consume them in moderation.

Here are the foods that may flare up your arthritis:

1 Sunflower oil

Sunflower oil can lead to joint pain and inflammation. Sunflower oil contains omega-6 fatty acids. Arachidonic acid (ARA), a polyunsaturated omega-6 fatty acid triggers the body to produce potent pro-inflammatory mediators such as prostaglandins and leukotrienes that cause inflammation - a key cause of arthritis pain.

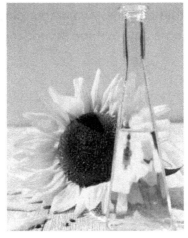

Polyunsaturated oils contain two types of essential fatty acids, omega-3 fatty acids, and omega-6 fatty acids. Your body itself cannot produce these fatty acids, so you need to get them from food. Omega-3 fats are anti-inflammatory, while omega-6 fats are pro-inflammatory. You need not completely stop taking omega-6 fatty acids. Both are essential for the body, but excess consumption of omega-6 fats is bad for rheumatoid arthritis. Avoid sunflower oil.

2. Sour curd

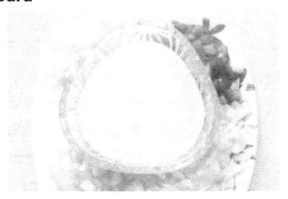

Freshly made curd in moderation may not be bad for arthritis, but sour curd often aggravates arthritis pain. Casein – a type of protein present in curd promote inflammation, which is the main reason for rheumatoid arthritis. Avoid sour curd; always eat fresh curd made on the same day, that too in moderation.

3. Tamarind

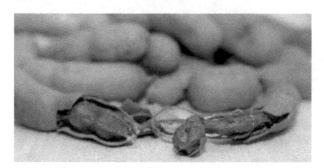

As such, tamarind is very beneficial for health but not for rheumatoid arthritis. This sweet and sour fruit can worsen arthritis pain and inflammation. Although studies suggest tamarind abrogates arthritis-mediated cartilage and bone degradation, but some people experience an increase in pain with tamarind. Again, the experience can differ from person to person; hence it is advised to observe your body's reaction to tamarind.

4. Nightshade vegetables

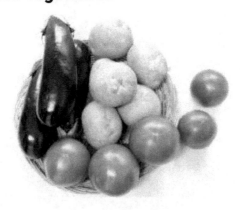

Both potatoes and eggplants are members of the nightshade family. Both contain the chemical solanine that plants use as a natural defense. It has a toxic effect on the body and can lead to gastrointestinal and neurological disorders. People claim that they experience arthritis pain and inflammation with nightshade vegetables, which can be due to solanine.

Other vegetables from the nightshade family are tomatoes and peppers. If you experience an increase in inflammation and pain after consuming any of these vegetables, avoid them. Even if you don't experience any pain, still eat them in moderation.

5. Black gram

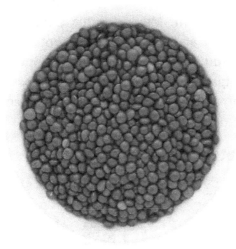

Black gram increases pro-inflammatory cytokines IL-1β and TNF-α and decreases anti-inflammatory cytokine IL-10. It means it increases inflammation in the body by increasing inflammation-causing protein and decreasing the protein that reduces inflammation in the body. Also, research suggests black gram decreases antioxidant effect in the body, which is more prominent in black gram without skin; boiling and not boiling the pulse doesn't have much difference in their effects.

6. Taro root/Arbi

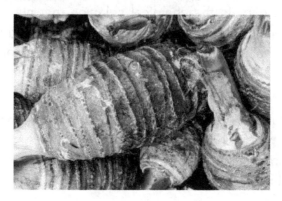

Taro root comprises of calcium oxalate in a needle-shaped crystal form, which can produce irritation and burning sensation when consumed in raw form. Many arthritis people claim that they experience swelling and pain after taro root consumption. They may cause the formation of kidney stones and gout (a type of arthritis), accompanied by some other health issues. Either avoid eating this root or boil the root for an extended period before cooking them.

7. Chilled water

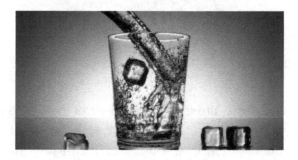

Chilled water can worsen autoimmune diseases, including rheumatoid arthritis. Chilled water causes constriction of blood vessels and reduces blood flow to the affected joint area. Due to reduced blood flow, the body's ability to clear out the impurities gets affected, and inflammation increases resulting in pain. Avoid drinking anything chill, whether it's a cold drink, iced tea, cold coffee, or plain chilled water.

8. Fried foods

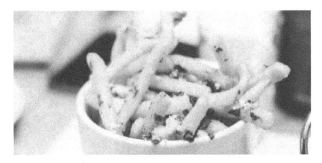

When foods are exposed to high temperatures, such as during frying, baking, barbecuing, and grilling, produce advanced glycation end product (AGE), which is a toxin. AGEs bind to RAGE (receptor for advanced glycation end-products) and activate pro-inflammatory cytokine production, thus become involved in inflammation and result in arthritis.

9. Processed foods and canned foods

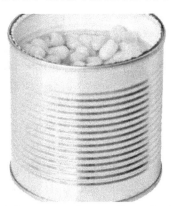

Canned foods contain excessive salt and other preservatives to achieve longer shelf lives. High sodium can increase inflammation in your body. Reducing salt consumption may help in reducing inflammation. Processed foods such as cakes, biscuit, and cheese contain hydrogenated oils that are high in trans fats, and trans fats trigger systemic inflammation. Avoid processed and canned foods to prevent arthritis.

10. Alcohol

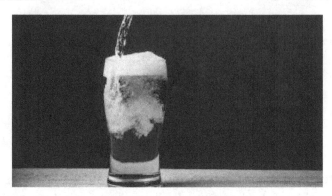

Drinking alcohol is injurious to health; you must have heard it many times. Alcohol may cause more inflammation, which can make symptoms of arthritis worse. Alcohol interferes with anti-inflammatory medicines that can increase your risk of stomach bleeding and ulcers and can be fatal. Never drink if you are on arthritis medication.

CONCLUSION

Not everyone reacts the same way to the foods mentioned above. Some can easily tolerate these foods, while others' pain gets worse. You know your body best. Observe yourself. Note down what you eat the whole day and observe if you experience an increase in pain, swelling, and inflammation. If any of the above foods were included in your diet, avoid eating them for about 1 to 2 weeks and see if your condition gets better. Just by avoiding these foods, preventing and managing your arthritis would be much easier. If you are young, healthy, and have no arthritis history in your family, limit your consumption of the foods mentioned above, and arthritis will never touch you in life.

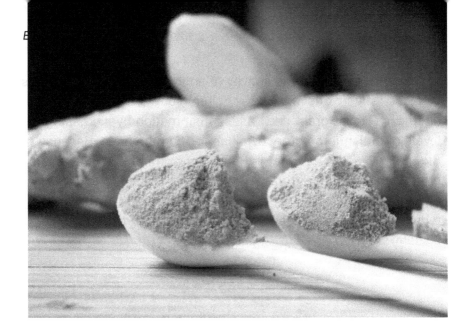

3.3

10 FOODS THAT HELP PREVENT AND CONTROL ARTHRITIS

To prevent and control arthritis, your diet should be rich in foods that have the following activities:
- Foods that reduce inflammation (omega-3 rich foods)
- Foods that have potent antioxidant property
- Foods that modulate immune activity
- Foods that balance the gut microbiome

Below are the 10 power foods that can prevent and treat arthritis naturally:

1. Horse gram

Horse gram is rich in polyphenols, flavonoids, and acts as an anti-inflammatory and an antioxidant. Studies show that horse gram significantly increases the activity of antioxidant enzymes such as catalase, superoxide dismutase, glutathione peroxidase, in liver and heart. Horse gram decreases inflammation by increasing the levels of anti-inflammatory cytokine IL-10 in the body. Because of the potent anti-inflammatory and antioxidant activities, horse gram can reverse arthritis. Additionally, it helps reduce body weight. Weight loss may help improve arthritis symptoms by reducing the excess load on your joints that cause pain and discomfort.

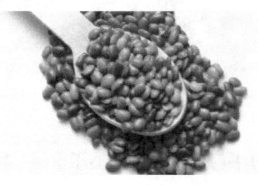

2. Turmeric

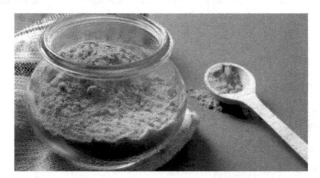

The main active ingredient in turmeric is curcumin. It is curcumin that gives turmeric bright yellow color. It produces potent anti-inflammatory and antioxidant effects. Typical medicines that are prescribed in arthritis are non-steroidal anti-inflammatory drugs (NSAIDs). These drugs work by inhibiting the activity of cyclooxygenase enzymes, COX-1, and COX-2. COX-1 is the good COX, while COX-2 is potentially troublesome. COX-1 synthesizes prostaglandins that help in maintaining the health of the stomach and intestine, while COX-2 synthesizes the inflammatory prostaglandins and oxygen-free radicals that enhance inflammation. These NSAIDs inhibit the COX-2 enzyme, but simultaneously they inhibit the good COX-1 too. Therefore, they may increase the risk of serious bowel and stomach side effects like ulcers and bleeding. Studies suggest curcumin has the chemical properties of a COX inhibitor and has no side effects like NSAIDs. Turmeric may help alleviate or prevent symptoms of arthritis. Turmeric is very effective in preventing arthritis.

Boil one glass of milk and add one tablespoon of turmeric powder in it. Drink it at night just before bed while it's still hot. In winter, eat plenty of fresh turmeric roots. They are more effective and beneficial than turmeric powder.

3. Ginger

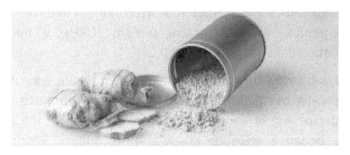

Ginger has potent antioxidant and anti-inflammatory properties. It increases the activities of antioxidant enzymes in the liver. Ginger contains phenolic compounds such as gingerol and shogaols as active components that protect body tissues against oxidative stress. Ginger also suppresses the synthesis of pro-inflammatory cytokines by suppressing NF-κB protein. It has been proven that ginger functions as a COX-2 inhibitor, just like NSAIDs, in controlling rheumatoid arthritis, osteoarthritis, and other types of arthritis. The anti-inflammatory properties of ginger help relieve pain and improve conditions in all types of arthritis.

4. Walnuts

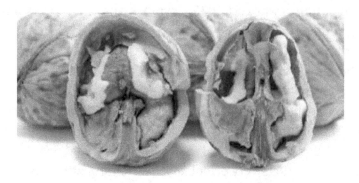

Walnuts have excellent antioxidant and anti-inflammatory activity. Phenolic content of walnut, especially in its skin, exhibits the highest ant-oxidative capacity. Walnuts are high in alpha-linolenic acid (ALA). They have the highest omega-3 content in comparison to other tree nuts. Omega-3 fats have anti-inflammatory effects that reduce inflammation. Elevated C-reactive protein (CRP) levels in the body indicate the inflammatory condition like RA. Studies show walnuts lower C-reactive protein (CRP), a marker of inflammation linked to arthritis.

Take a handful of walnut kernels or two whole walnuts, soak them in water overnight. Eat them on an empty stomach the next morning. Soaking is an important step, especially in the summer season, because walnuts are warm in nature. Walnuts can produce heat in the body and can cause mouth ulcers if you consume them without soaking.

5. Extra virgin olive oil

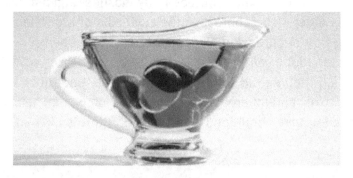

Extra virgin olive oil is rich in Omega-3 fatty acids. Omega-3 fats work as an anti-inflammatory and help reduce pain and swelling in arthritic joints. Alongside Omega-3 fatty acids, olive oil also contains oleocanthal, a natural compound that has scientifically proven to produce similar pain-relieving results as non-steroidal anti-inflammatory drugs (NSAIDs). Oleocanthal works in a similar way to NSAIDs by inhibiting the same enzyme responsible for inflammation and pain. Additionally, phenolic compounds present in extra virgin olive oil reduce cartilage degradation, bone erosion, and joint edema.

Also, a recent study suggests applying topical extra virgin olive oil is effective in controlling of inflammatory pain of joints in rheumatic arthritis.

Among all types of olive oils, extra virgin olive oil exhibits maximum health benefits, because it is the least processed or refined type. It contains maximum phenolic antioxidants and oleocanthal content.

6. Licorice root

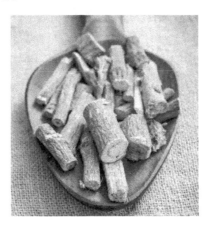

Licorice decreases the levels of pro-inflammatory cytokines. Glycyrrhizin is the component in licorice, which exhibits an anti-inflammatory effect by mimicking the actions of steroids in the body. Furthermore, licorice prevents oxidative damages. Licorice increases the availability of cortisol in the body by preventing the body from using up its stores of cortisol; it reduces the conversion of cortisol to inactive cortisone. Cortisol can help reduce inflammation, also, suppresses the immune system, easing the pain and occurrence of arthritis. Be aware that licorice can cause anxiety and high blood pressure. If you are on medication of blood pressure, diabetes or diuretics, don't use licorice, it may interfere with the drug's efficacy. Consult your doctor before taking licorice. Women who are pregnant are not advised to take licorice root in any form. Licorice should be taken under medical advice. Roasting licorice roots increase their anti-inflammatory activity. Research show roasted licorice may inhibit the acute inflammation more potently. The best way to take licorice root is to roast it, crush it and to boil up the root in order to make a herbal tea.

7. Flax seeds

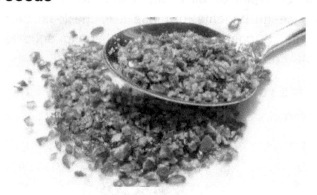

Flax seeds are also known as linseeds. Flax seeds and flax seeds oil are rich in alpha-linolenic acid (ALA), an omega-3 fatty acid that helps decrease inflammation and joint pain in arthritis. Phytochemicals called lignans found in flax seeds oil have anti-inflammatory and antioxidant properties that help reduce the risk of arthritis. Flax seeds are also rich in fiber that helps to ease bowel movement combating constipation and keeping the digestive system healthy.

Use dry roasted and ground flax seeds instead of whole to help your body get the most nutrients from flax seeds for rheumatoid arthritis. This step is necessary to increase their absorption.

Whole flax seeds are not easily digestible as their outer shell is hard for the intestines to break down, eating ground flax seeds increase the absorption of the nutrients. Whole flax seeds are chemically stable, but ground flax seeds may go rancid when left exposed to air at room temperature for a longer period, because of oxidation. The best way is to roast and grind them just before the use, to prevent oxidation and increase absorption.

**Read 10 power foods to get rid of anemia in the book "Eat So What! The Power of Vegetarianism."

8. Spinach

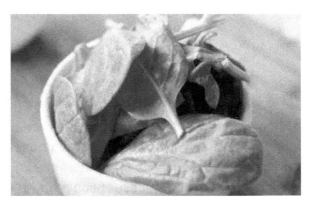

Vitamin K is a crucial nutrient for joint health. Your body needs vitamin K for healthy bone growth and repair. Lack of vitamin K in the body can increase the risk of osteoarthritis. Spinach is rich in vitamin K, which can help with inflammation caused by arthritis. Spinach is high in bone-preserving calcium. Free radical compounds can destroy healthy cells in the body, and antioxidants destroy those free radicals. Spinach is an excellent source of fiber and antioxidants like vitamins A, C, and E, which protect cells from free radical damage and help reduce inflammation.

Spinach is especially high in the antioxidant kaempferol, an important phytochemical that can bring down the levels of the inflammatory cytokine. Kaempferol inhibits several enzymes that induce oxidative stress that cause rheumatoid arthritis. Study

131

shows kaempferol reduces inflammation and prevents the progression of osteoarthritis. Start adding spinach in your diet to prevent or control arthritis. Avoid eating raw spinach, instead, sauté or blanch them before use. Cooking spinach increases its nutrition value. Also, add 1 tablespoon of lemon juice while blanching. Eating spinach with vitamin C boosts your iron absorption, which exhibits other health benefits.

9. Prebiotic

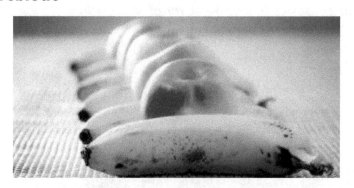

It is well known that a high-fat diet doubles the body fat percentage and causes obesity. Osteoarthritis in obese people is assumed to be a consequence of undue stress on joints. Researchers have found that obese people have more pro-inflammatory bacteria and almost completely lacked certain beneficial, probiotic bacteria in their guts compared to lean people. This causes inflammation throughout their body, leading to very rapid joint deterioration. These pro-inflammatory bacteria in the gut, which are governed by diet – could be the key driving force behind osteoarthritis. A high-fat diet influences the gut bacteria negatively, allowing harmful bacteria to overgrow. Compared to lean people, osteoarthritis progresses much more quickly in obese people.

Prebiotics are plant fibers. These fibers aren't digestible by humans, so they pass through the digestive system, where they act as fertilizers. They become food for the bacteria and other microbes in the gut and stimulate the growth of healthy bacteria, like Bifidobacteria. The regular consumption of prebiotics foods increases the good bacteria in gut and crowd out bad ones, like pro-inflammatory bacteria. This, in turn, decreases systemic inflammation and slows cartilage breakdown. While prebiotic foods don't reduce obesity, it completely reverses the other symptoms related to arthritis, making the joints more movable. Some examples of prebiotics are banana, apple (don't remove the skin as the skin contains most prebiotic benefits), onion, garlic, oats, asparagus, and yams.

10. Water

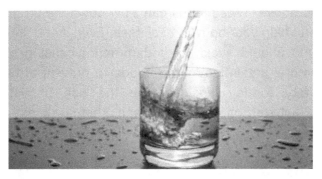

Dehydration can make symptoms of arthritis worse. Your joints need fluids to move smoothly. If you are dehydrated, it affects your joints mobility too. Lack of hydration produces friction between the contact point of the joint. Over time, dry cartilage may die and peel from their contact surface of the bones. Drinking more water can improve your arthritis condition for several reasons: water helps to fight inflammation by flushing toxins out of the body. When the joints move, they pull water from the bone marrow to the joint cavity and provides lubrication. If there is not enough water, the joints can't move as they should. Also, water can stimulate the production of synovial fluid that lubricates and cushions the joints and cartilage surrounding them. This keeps the bones from rubbing together, reduces inflammation around the joint, and encourages the growth of new cells in the cartilage tissues. So, increase your water intake to reduce the pain associated with arthritis. For proper lubrication and to control painful symptoms, it is important to drink between two to three liters of water every day, which equals to 8 to 12 glasses of water.

CONCLUSION

Arthritis is no longer a disease of old age. People, even in their late 30s, have started seeing the symptoms of arthritis. The reasons are unhealthy foods that promote inflammation in the body, lack of sunlight exposure, and a diet deficient in anti-inflammatory foods. People who have arthritis can effectively reduce symptoms and inflammation associated with arthritis with the foods mentioned above. These foods can slow down the progression of arthritis and help your body to heal itself. Even if you are a healthy person, you should avoid the inflammation-causing foods and include natural anti-inflammatory foods to prevent arthritis. Anti-inflammatory foods also decrease the risk of autoimmune disorders, diabetes, obesity, cancer, and other diseases.

KEY POINTS

✓ Pain and inflammation are more prominent in the wet season.

✓ Avoid sour food.

✓ Limit your nightshade vegetables.

✓ Eat more omega-3 rich food.

✓ It is important to empty bowel frequently. Constipation aggravates arthritis, pain, and inflammation.

✓ Avoid cold breeze.

✓ Take a hot shower every day. It reduces stiffness by stimulating blood flow to frozen joints and stiff muscles.

✓ Add antioxidant spices to your diet.

3

DIET PLAN

Diet Plan for

Healthy and disease-free Life

Diabetes

Hypertension

Arthritis

Diabetes + Hypertension

Hypertension + Arthritis

Diabetes + Arthtitis

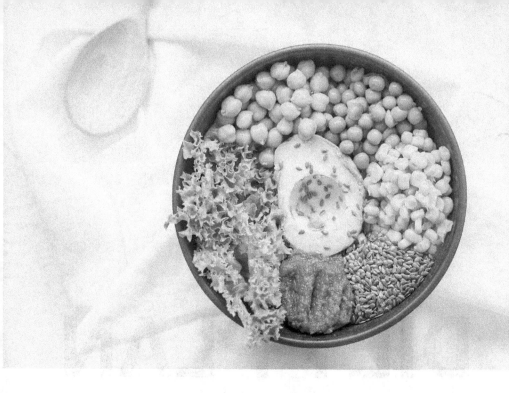

DIET PLAN FOR HEALTHY AND DISEASE-FREE LIFE

- Drink lemon water on an empty stomach.

- Eat overnight soaked dry fruits every day.

    - In winter, 8 almonds + 6 cashews + 6 pistachios + 8 raisins + 2 figs + 4 dates.

    - In summer, (Must be soaked overnight) 5-6 almonds + 4 cashews + 4 pistachios + 4 raisins + 1 fig + 2 dates.

- Drink green tea with lemon juice. If you must add sugar, then add jaggery powder instead of sugar in it.

- Add barley flour to your whole wheat flour in a ratio of 1:7. Add 1 kg barley flour in 7 kg of whole wheat flour.

- Drink more water. Water helps remove toxins from your blood through urine.

- Eat one crushed garlic on an empty stomach once in a week.

- Crush fenugreek seeds and use fenugreek powder in cooking. Fenugreek seeds are bitter in taste, so add 1-2 teaspoon only. If you can tolerate the bitter taste, then add up to 1 tablespoon.

- Use spices such as turmeric, cinnamon, and cumin in cooking.

- Eat one flax seeds laddoo every day.

- Use cold-pressed oil in cooking, such as mustard oil instead of refined oil.

- Use three types of oil- mustard oil for cooking, refined oil such as soybean oil for deep frying, and extra virgin olive oil for sautéing or low flame cooking. Don't use olive oil to deep fry.

- Eat a variety of sprouts.

- Eat seasonal fruits and vegetables, eat them in plenty in season avoid eating non-seasonal fruits and vegetables; they are inferior in nutritional content.

- Drink one glass of milk daily no matter what's your age. Milk is not only required for kids, it is a must for all age groups.

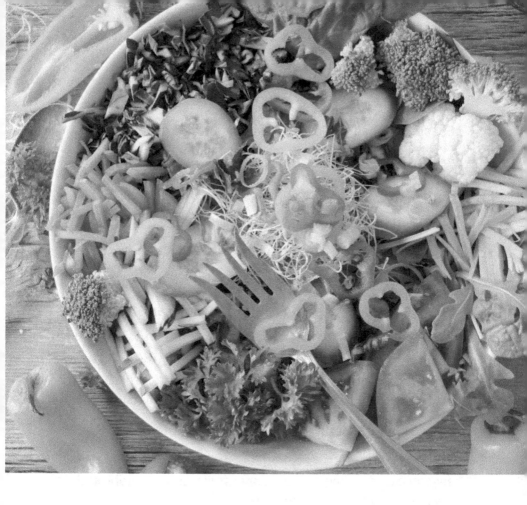

DIET PLAN TO CONTROL DIABETES

✓ Soak one tablespoon of fenugreek seeds overnight in 250 ml of water. The next morning chew these seeds and drink the fenugreek water. Do this every day (highly effective).

✓ Chew some (3-4) basil leaves or add them in your morning green tea.

✓ Eat a handful of overnight soaked nuts.

✓ Replace potatoes with sweet potatoes and white rice with brown rice.

✓ Eat one crushed garlic on an empty stomach thrice a week. (after one hour of having soaked fenugreek seeds).

✓ Add barley flour to your whole wheat flour in a ratio of 1:7. Add 1 kg barley flour in 7 kg of whole wheat flour. Beta-glucan of barley is very effective in preventing diabetes and also prevent weight gain.

✓ Drink more water, about 2-3 liters, equivalent to 10 -12 glass of 250 ml. Water helps remove excess sugar from your blood through urine, and it helps prevent dehydration.

✓ In season, drink 50 ml to 100 ml of fresh bitter gourd juice every day. Cook bitter gourd with its peel. Don't remove the skin.

✓ Eat a variety of sprouts every day.

✓ Add flax seeds in your dough or add them in yogurt.

✓ Eat vegetables that have high water content such as bottle gourd and ridge gourd.

✓ Eat non-starchy vegetables such as carrot, cabbage, cauliflower, green beans, and broccoli.

✓ Eat vitamin C foods such as amla, lemon, orange, and capsicum.

✓ Use olive oil, canola oil, and mustard oil in cooking.

✓ Include apple, oatmeal, and beans in your diet for high soluble fiber.

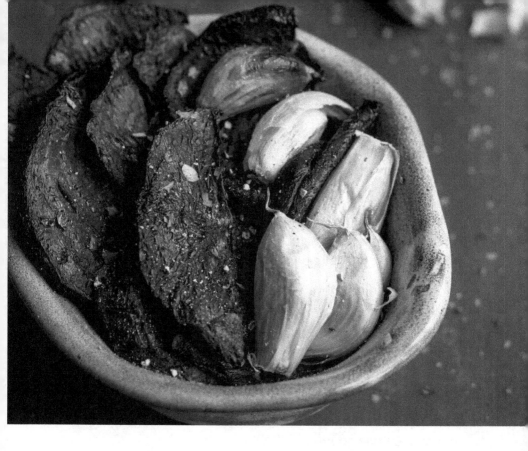

DIET PLAN TO CONTROL HYPERTENSION

✓ Add one tablespoon of honey in warm lemon water and drink it on an empty stomach.

✓ Eat one crushed garlic on an empty stomach every day (if you experience mouth ulcer or heat in the body, reduce the frequency to 5 times a week).

✓ Soak one tablespoon of fenugreek seeds overnight in 250 ml of water. The next morning chew these seeds and drink the fenugreek water. Do this thrice a week.

✓ Drink green tea and add lemon to it.

✓ Eat a handful of overnight soaked nuts.

✓ Eat one banana every day, especially if you are taking hypertension medicines.

✓ In season, eat multigrain beetroot paratha. Have 50 to 100 ml of beetroot juice every day.

✓ Add barley flour to your whole wheat flour in a ratio of 2:10. Add 200 gm of barley flour to 1 kg of whole wheat flour. Beta-glucan of barley is very effective in preventing hypertension and prevent weight gain.

✓ In winter, eat plenty of spinach, kale, and chenopodium (bathua).

✓ Eat one flax seeds laddoo every day.

✓ Eat plenty of sweet potatoes, especially the purple-fleshed sweet potatoes.

✓ Eat plenty of legumes such as lentils, chickpeas, kidney beans, and soybeans for potassium, magnesium, and fiber.

✓ Drink plenty of water, especially on the day you consume more salt.

✓ Eat fresh fruits, like apples, oranges, and bananas.

✓ Drink low-fat cow's milk boiled with turmeric powder every night.

✓ Eat mixed veg raita with lunch.

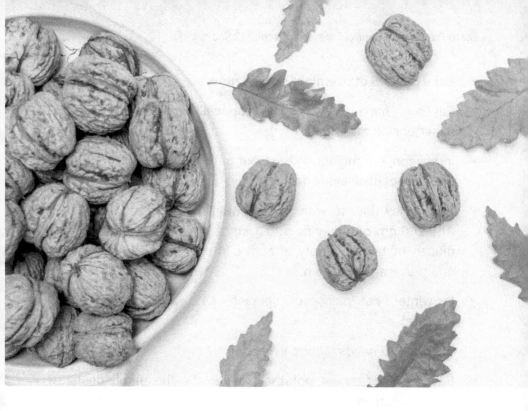

DIET PLAN TO CONTROL ARTHRITIS

- ✓ Take a handful of walnut kernels or two whole walnuts, and two dried figs soaked in water overnight. Eat them on an empty stomach in the morning. Do this every day.

- ✓ Eat horse gram (kulthi) as much as possible. Make horse gram dal or powder it and use with your whole wheat flour or add the powder in buttermilk.

- ✓ In winter, eat plenty of fresh turmeric roots.

- ✓ Drink low-fat cow's milk boiled with turmeric powder at night.

- ✓ Eat low-fat plain yogurt.

- ✓ Drink green tea mixed with freshly crushed ginger.

✓ Use canola oil or mustard oil in cooking, avoid sunflower oil and corn oil, which are rich in omega-6 fats.

✓ Eat sprouted horse gram along with sprouted mung bean, and black chickpeas.

✓ Eat a handful of soaked nuts, including walnuts, pistachios, almonds, and figs.

✓ Increase your soybean consumption. Add soybean flour to your whole wheat flour in a ratio of 1:10. Add 1kg of soybean flour to 10 kg of whole wheat flour.

✓ Eat one flax seeds laddoo every day.

✓ Eat one crushed garlic on an empty stomach thrice a week.

✓ Eat plenty of green vegetables including, spinach, kale, and fenugreek leaves.

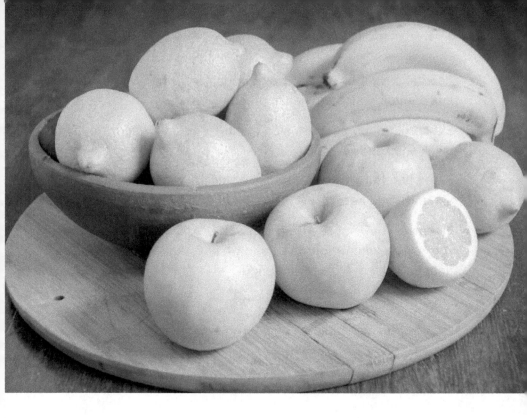

DIET PLAN TO CONTROL DIABETES + HYPERTENSION

✓ Drink warm lemon water on an empty stomach.

✓ After half an hour, eat soaked fenugreek seeds and drink the fenugreek water. Do this every day.

✓ After one hour, eat one crushed garlic. Do this every day.

✓ Have green tea with added lemon and basil leaves.

✓ Eat a handful of overnight soaked nuts.

✓ Drink about 2-3 liters of water in a day.

✓ Add barley flour to your whole wheat flour in a ratio of 2:10. Add 200 gm of barley flour to 1 kg of whole wheat flour.

- ✓ Eat one banana, especially if you are taking hypertension medicines. Don't remove the banana from your diet just because you have diabetes. Cut the sugar intake in tea and other high glycemic fruits.

- ✓ In season, drink 50 ml to 100 ml of fresh bitter gourd juice every day.

- ✓ In season, eat multigrain beetroot paratha. Have 50 to 100 ml of beetroot juice every day.

- ✓ Eat sprouts every day.

- ✓ Add flax seeds in dough or add them in a yogurt fruit salad.

- ✓ Eat bottle gourd, carrot, and ridge gourd.

- ✓ Replace potatoes with sweet potatoes and eat them in moderation.

- ✓ Drink low-fat cow's milk boiled with turmeric powder at night.

- ✓ Eat plenty of spinach, kale, cabbage, and chenopodium (bathua).

- ✓ Increase legumes consumption, including lentils, chickpeas, kidney beans, and soybeans.

- ✓ Eat vitamin C foods such as amla, lemon, orange, and capsicum.

- ✓ Use olive oil, canola oil, and mustard oil in cooking.

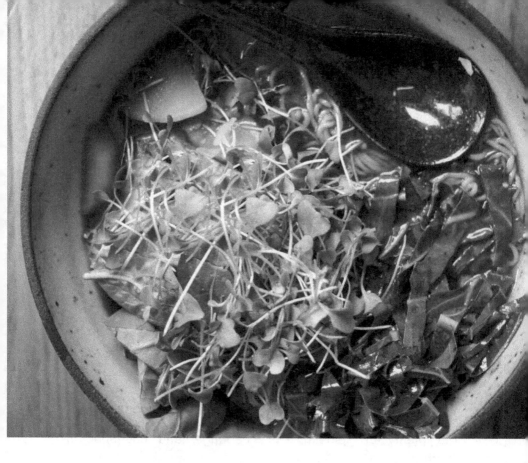

DIET PLAN TO CONTROL HYPERTENSION + ARTHRITIS

- ✓ Eat one crushed garlic on an empty stomach every day (if you experience mouth ulcer or heat in the body, reduce the frequency to 5 times a week).

- ✓ After half an hour, eat soaked fenugreek seeds and drink the fenugreek water. Do this thrice a week.

- ✓ Drink green tea mixed with freshly crushed ginger.

✓ Eat a handful of overnight soaked dry fruits, including two walnuts, two dried figs, five almonds, four cashew nuts, four pistachios, and four raisins. Eat them daily.

✓ Drink low-fat turmeric milk at night.

✓ Eat one banana every day, especially if you are taking hypertension medicines.

✓ Add barley flour and soybean flour to your whole wheat flour in a ratio 2:1:10. Add 200 gm of barley flour and 100 gm of soybean flour in 1 kg of whole wheat flour.

✓ Eat plenty of horse gram (kulthi). Make horse gram dal or powder it and use with your whole wheat flour or add the powder in buttermilk.

✓ In season, eat multigrain beetroot paratha. Have 50 to 100 ml of beetroot juice every day.

✓ In winter, eat plenty of fresh turmeric roots, spinach, kale, fenugreek leaves, chenopodium, and sweet potatoes, especially the purple-fleshed sweet potatoes.

✓ Eat one flax seeds laddoo every day.

✓ Eat mixed veg raita with lunch.

✓ Eat plenty of legumes such as lentils, chickpeas, kidney beans, and soybeans for potassium, magnesium, and fiber.

✓ Drink plenty of water, especially on the day you consume more salt.

✓ Use extra virgin olive oil (only for shallow fry), canola oil or mustard oil in cooking, avoid sunflower oil and corn oil, which are rich in omega-6 fats.

✓ Eat fresh fruits, like apples, oranges, and bananas.

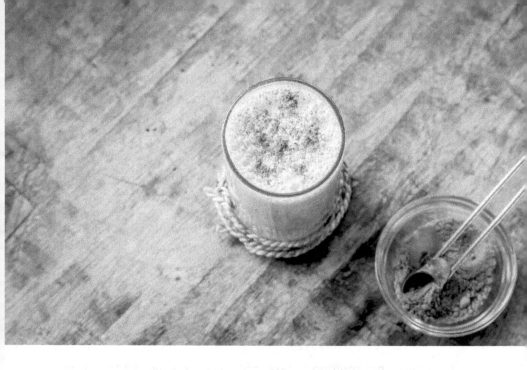

DIET PLAN TO CONTROL DIABETES + ARTHRITIS

✓ Soak one tablespoon of fenugreek seeds overnight in 250 ml of water. The next morning chew these seeds and drink the fenugreek water. Do this every day. (highly effective)

✓ Eat a handful of overnight soaked walnuts and dried figs (2 pieces). Eat them daily.

✓ Drink green tea mixed with crushed ginger and basil leaves (3-4 leaves).

✓ Eat one crushed garlic on an empty stomach thrice a week (after one hour of having soaked fenugreek seeds).

✓ Add barley flour and soybean flour to your whole wheat flour in a ratio of 1.5:1:10. Add 1.5 kg barley flour and 1 kg of soybean flour in 10 kg of whole wheat flour.

✓ Replace potatoes with sweet potatoes and white rice with brown rice.

✓ Drink 2-3 liters of water in a day.

✓ Add horse gram (kulthi) in your diet.

✓ In winter, eat plenty of fresh turmeric roots. Drink low-fat cow's milk boiled with turmeric powder at night.

✓ In season, drink 50 ml to 100 ml of fresh bitter gourd juice every day. Cook bitter gourd with its peel. Don't remove the skin.

✓ Eat sprouted horse gram, sprouted mung bean, and black chickpeas.

✓ Add flax seeds in dough or add them in the yogurt fruit salad.

✓ Eat vegetables that have high water content such as bottle gourd and ridge gourd.

✓ Eat non-starchy vegetables such as carrot, cabbage, cauliflower, green beans, and broccoli.

✓ Eat plenty of green vegetables including, spinach, kale, and fenugreek leaves.

✓ Use olive oil, canola oil, and mustard oil in cooking, and avoid sunflower oil and corn oil.

✓ Include apple, oatmeal, and beans in your diet for high soluble fiber.

REFERENCES

1. Soheil Z, Habsah A, "A Review on Antibacterial, Antiviral, and Antifungal Activity of Curcumin." Biomed Res Int. 2014; 2014: 186864.
2. Silagy C, Neil A, "Garlic as a lipid lowering agent--a meta-analysis." R Coll Physicians Lond. Jan-Feb 1994;28(1):39-45.
3. Matthias B, Mandy S, "Fiber and magnesium intake and incidence of type 2 diabetes: a prospective study and meta-analysis." Arch Intern Med. 2007 May 14;167(9):956-65.
4. Karin R, Toben C, Fakler P, "Effect of garlic on serum lipids: an updated meta-analysis." Nutr Rev. 2013 May;71(5):282-99.
5. Holly L, Sharon A, "Garlic and onions: Their cancer prevention properties." Cancer Prev Res (Phila). 2015 Mar; 8(3): 181–189.
6. Ranade M, Mudgalkar N, "A simple dietary addition of fenugreek seed leads to the reduction in blood glucose levels: A parallel-group, randomized single-blind trial." Ayu. 2017 Jan-Jun; 38(1-2): 24–27.
7. Calado A, Neves M, "The Effect of Flaxseed in Breast Cancer: A Literature Review." Front Nutr. 2018; 5: 4.
8. Chikako M, Taeko K, "Effects of glycolipids from spinach on mammalian DNA polymerases." Biochem Pharmacol. 2003 Jan 15;65(2):259-67.
9. Mondal S, Varma S, "Double-blinded randomized controlled trial for immunomodulatory effects of Tulsi (Ocimum sanctum Linn.) leaf extract on healthy volunteers." Ethnopharmacol. 2011 Jul 14;136(3):452-
10. Dokania M, Kishore K, Sharma PK, "Effect of Ocimum sanctum extract on sodium nitrite-induced experimental amnesia in mice." Thai J Pharma Sci. 2011; 35:123.
11. Eddouks M, Amina B, "Antidiabetic plants improving insulin sensitivity." J Pharm Pharmacol. 2014 Sep;66(9):1197-214.
12. Widjaja S, Rusdiana, "Glucose Lowering Effect of Basil Leaves in Diabetic Rats." J Med Sci. 2019 May 15; 7(9): 1415–1417.
13. Gallagher J, Vinod Yalamanchili V, "The Effect of Vitamin D on Calcium Absorption in Older Women." J Clin Endocrinol Metab. 2012 Oct; 97(10): 3550.
14. Gupta R, Gangoliya S, "Reduction of phytic acid and enhancement of bioavailable micronutrients in food grains." J Food Sci Technol. 2015 Feb; 52(2): 676–684.
15. Lee A, Thurnham D, "Consumption of tomato products with olive oil but not sunflower oil increases the antioxidant activity of plasma." Free Radical Biol Med. 2000 Nov 15;29(10):1051-5.
16. Malouf M, Grimley E, "Folic acid with or without vitamin B12 for cognition and dementia." Cochrane Database Syst Rev, 2003;(4): CD004514.
17. Abularrage C, Sidawy A, "Effect of folic Acid and vitamins B6 and B12 on microcirculatory vasoreactivity in patients with hyperhomocysteinemia." Vasc Endovascular Surg. 2007 Aug-Sep;41(4):339-45.
18. Sarwar N, Gao P, "Diabetes mellitus, fasting blood glucose concentration, and risk of vascular disease: a collaborative meta-analysis of 102 prospective studies. Emerging Risk Factors Collaboration." Lancet. 2010; 26; 375:2215-2222.
19. Bourne R, Stevens G, "Causes of vision loss worldwide, 1990-2010: a systematic analysis." Lancet Global Health 2013;1:e339-e349
20. "Diabetes facts & figures." The International Diabetes Federation (IDF), 2020, https://www.idf.org/aboutdiabetes/what-is-diabetes/facts-figures.html
21. Cruz K, Oliveira A, "Antioxidant role of zinc in diabetes mellitus." World J Diabetes. 2015 Mar 15; 6(2): 333–337.

22. Abdelsalam S, Hesham M, "The Role of Protein Tyrosine Phosphatase (PTP)-1B in Cardiovascular Disease and Its Interplay with Insulin Resistance." Biomolecules. 2019 Jul; 9(7): 286.

23. Alam MD, Uddin R, "Beneficial Role of Bitter Melon Supplementation in Obesity and Related Complications in Metabolic Syndrome." J Lipids; 2015: 496169.

24. Padmaja Chaturvedi P, "Antidiabetic potentials of Momordica charantia: multiple mechanisms behind the effects." J Med Food. 2012 Feb;15(2):101-7.

25. Joseph B, Jini D, "Antidiabetic effects of Momordica charantia (bitter melon) and its medicinal potency." Asian Pac J Trop Dis. 2013 Apr; 3(2): 93–102.

26. Tayyab F, Lal S, "Medicinal plants and its impact on diabetes." World J Pharm Res. 2012;1(4):1019–1046.

27. Paul A, Raychaudhuri S, "Medicinal uses and molecular identification of two Momordica charantia varieties - a review." E J Bio. 2010;6(2):43–51.

28. Garg A, "High-monounsaturated-fat diets for patients with diabetes mellitus: a meta-analysis." Am J Clin Nutr, 1998 Mar;67(3 Suppl):577S-582S.

29. Kassaian N, Azadbakht L, "Effect of fenugreek seeds on blood glucose and lipid profiles in type 2 diabetic patients." Int J Vitam Nutr Res. 2009 Jan;79(1):34-9.

30. Kesika P, Sivamaruthi B, "Do Probiotics Improve the Health Status of Individuals with Diabetes Mellitus? A Review on Outcomes of Clinical Trials." Biomed Res Int. 2019; 2019: 1531567.

31. D'souza J, D'souza P, "Anti-diabetic effects of the Indian indigenous fruit Emblica Officinalis Gaertn: active constituents and modes of action." Food Funct. 2014 Apr;5(4):635-44.

32. Sharabi K, Tavares C, "Molecular Pathophysiology of Hepatic Glucose Production," Mol Aspects Med. 2015 Dec; 46: 21–33.

33. Santhi K, Rajamani S, "Amla, a Marvelous Fruit for Type -2 Diabetics-A Review." Int. J. Curr. Microbiol. App. Sci. 2017, 5:116-123

34. Radzeviciene L, Ostrauskas R, "Adding Salt to Meals as a Risk Factor of Type 2 Diabetes Mellitus: A Case–Control Study." Nutrients. 2017 Jan; 9(1): 67.

35. Kato Y, Domoto T, "Effect on Blood Pressure of Daily Lemon Ingestion and Walking." J Nutr Metab. 2014; 2014: 912684.

36. Dehkordi F, Kamkhah A, "Antihypertensive effect of Nigella sativa seed extract in patients with mild hypertension." Fundam Clin Pharmacol, 2008 Aug;22(4):447.

37. Diego A, Ocampo B, "Dietary Nitrate from Beetroot Juice for Hypertension: A Systematic Review." Biomolecules. 2018 Dec; 8(4): 134.

38. Ried K, Fakler P, "Potential of garlic (Allium sativum) in lowering high blood pressure: mechanisms of action and clinical relevance." Integr Blood Press Control. 2014; 7: 71–82.

39. Aluko E, Olubobokun T, "Honey's Ability to Reduce Blood Pressure and Heart Rate in Healthy Male Subjects." Frontiers in Science, 2014

40. Jovanovski E, Bosco L, "Effect of Spinach, a High Dietary Nitrate Source, on Arterial Stiffness and Related Hemodynamic Measures: A Randomized, Controlled Trial in Healthy Adults." Clin Nutr Res. 2015 Jul; 4(3): 160–167.

41. Hekmatpou D, Mortaji S, "The Effectiveness of Olive Oil in Controlling Morning Inflammatory Pain of Phalanges and Knees Among Women with Rheumatoid Arthritis: A Randomized Clinical Trial." Rehabil Nurs. Mar/Apr 2020;45(2):106.

42. Rajagopal V, Pushpan C, "Comparative effect of horse gram and black gram on inflammatory mediators and antioxidant," Journal of Food and Drug Analysis, 2017, Pages 845-853

43. Huang Q, Mao-Jie Wang M, "Can active components of licorice, glycyrrhizin and glycyrrhetinic acid, lick rheumatoid arthritis." Oncotarget, 2016 Jan: 1193–1202.

IMPORTANT TERMINOLOGY

Arteries: Arteries are blood vessels that carry oxygen-rich blood from the heart to the body.

Vascular: Vascular is related to vessels that carry blood in the body.

Vasoconstriction: Vaso means vessels, so vasoconstriction means narrowing of the blood vessels.

Vasodilation: Dilation or widening of blood vessels.

Glucose: Glucose means sweet in Greek. It is a type of sugar. You get carbohydrates from foods, which break down into glucose, and your body uses it for energy.

Hyperglycemia: Hyperglycemia refers to high levels of sugar (glucose) in the blood.

Bioavailability: The actual proportion of a substance that reaches the blood circulation after it introduced into the body to show its effect.

Free radicals: Free radicals are the unpaired electrons that form due to the oxidative process in the body. These unpaired electrons like to be in pairs, so they pair with the electrons in proteins and DNA and damage them.

Antioxidants: Body has antioxidants, which neutralize free radicals by inhibiting the oxidative process that forms free radicals.

Oxidative stress: When free radicals outnumber the naturally occurring antioxidants, it results in oxidative stress. This imbalance leads to cell and tissue damage, including DNA, protein, and lipids. Damage to your DNA increases your risk of chronic diseases such as cancer, rheumatoid arthritis, diabetics, stroke, and aging.

Inflammation: Inflammation is the response of the body to harmful pathogens, and irritants, and eliminate the initial cause of cell injury. Body releases white blood cells to heal the damaged cells. When the immune system mistakenly attacks healthy tissue, it causes harmful abnormal inflammation. Reasons for abnormal inflammation are stress, smoking, and alcohol consumption. Some examples of diseases associated with abnormal inflammations are rheumatoid arthritis, psoriasis, and inflammatory bowel diseases.

ABBREVIATIONS

RA- Rheumatoid Arthritis

BP- Blood pressure

LDL- Low-density lipoproteins

HDL- High-density lipoprotein

COX- Cyclooxygenase

PG- Prostaglandin

RAAS- Renin–angiotensin–aldosterone syste

EAT TO PREVENT AND CONTROL DISEASE
Cookbook

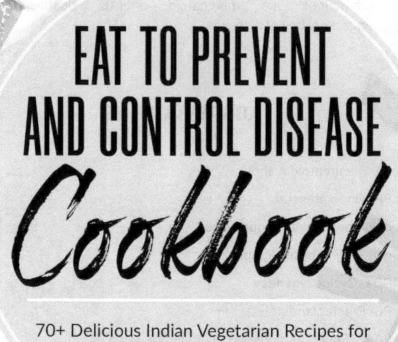

70+ Delicious Indian Vegetarian Recipes for
Healthy Living with Dedicated Recipes
for Diabetes, Hypertension,
and Arthritis

LA FONCEUR

EAT

TO **PREVENT**

AND **CONTROL**

DISEASE

COOKBOOK

70+ Delicious Indian Vegetarian Recipes for Healthy Living
with Dedicated Recipes for Diabetes, Hypertension, and
Arthritis

LA FONCEUR

Eb

emerald books

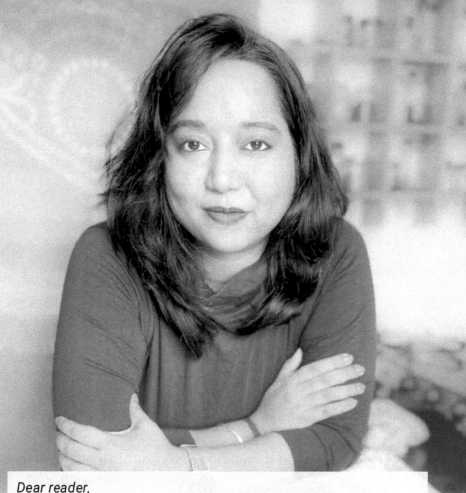

Dear reader,

The aim of **Eat to Prevent and Control Disease Cookbook** is to help you incorporate superfoods into your diet in such a way that they become part of your regular diet, and you eat them for the taste, not just for health. This cookbook brings you delicious recipes of superfoods that can help you prevent and manage chronic diseases.

Masters of Pharmacy,
Research Scientist,
Registered Pharmacist

ACKNOWLEDGEMENTS

A special thanks to my family for sharing the load of preparing this cookbook with me. This cookbook wouldn't have been possible without the help of my mom, who perfected all the cooking techniques and fundamentals while I was developing the recipes. Special thanks to my sister for giving me the technical help and moral support to make this cookbook with complete focus. Last but not least, thanks to my dad for always encouraging me to push my limits.

INTRODUCTION

Whether it's the laboratory or the kitchen, it's all about experimenting until you reach the perfect formulation! Not much difference.

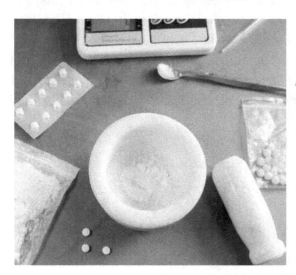

From making a perfect formulation in a mortar and pestle

To make the perfect spice blend in mortar and pestle

It's all about the correct technique! Not much difference.

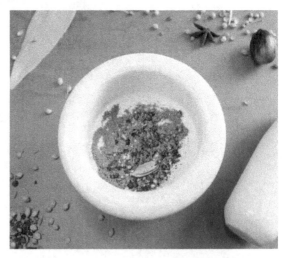

From following SOPs to following recipes, it's all about the experience that comes from practice. Basics are the same.

The specialty of Indian cooking is that even if you give the same ingredients and the same recipe to different people, the taste of the food prepared by them will be different in all. This is because of the spices involved in Indian cooking. Spices contain volatile oils that give them a distinctive aroma and taste. All spices contain volatile oils, and the roasting and cooking method helps the spices release volatile oils. The amount of volatile oil released can increase or decrease the flavor of food. The way you cook, the cooking time, even the type of flame, low, medium, or high, can all affect the taste of the food. You just need to know the right technique which will make the food most delicious. In this cookbook, you will learn all the techniques to make your food flavorsome. Once you master the techniques, you can start experimenting and doing some additions and omissions in the recipes as per your taste.

Everyone's taste is different. Some like to eat spicy while some prefer mild. Some like to eat gravy, some like dry, and some like curry. All these tastes have been taken care of in this cookbook. You will find all types of food like gravy, dry, and curry in the cookbook, and the spiciness is kept medium. You can adjust the spiciness according to your taste. Apart from this, healthy sweets, snacks, beverages, and tangy dishes are also included in the cookbook, which are delicious as well as nutritious.

Make from scratch! No short cuts

Indian cooking requires very few store-bought items, and the ones that are required can be easily made at home. You will be surprised to know how easily your store-bought items can be made at home. All the recipes in this cookbook are made from scratch. These simple and cost-effective ways can have a tremendous positive impact on your health.

This cookbook brings you delicious ways to incorporate superfoods into your diet that are discussed in *Eat to Prevent and Control Disease*.

The cookbook is completely based on superfoods. Each recipe in this cookbook includes one or more superfoods. In the book *Eat to Prevent and Control Disease*, you learned about the powerful superfoods you should be eating every day. But adding them to your diet doesn't have to be boring. You don't need to eat them forcefully just for the sake of health. This cookbook brings you many delicious and mouth-watering recipes of superfoods that you can eat anytime, any day. These dishes will satisfy your taste buds as well as strengthen your immunity and protect you from chronic diseases with their therapeutic effects.

Eat to Prevent and Control Disease Cookbook is divided into 7 parts, each with different sets of superfood recipes. You will find out how you can boost your immunity with delicious foods.

Certain foods become more nutritious when combined with other foods because they increase the absorption of nutrients into the bloodstream, giving you maximum health benefits. This cookbook provides several tempting recipes for combining the ideal nutrients so that you can get the maximum health benefits from them.

This cookbook has dedicated recipes for diabetes, high blood pressure, and arthritis. You'll learn how to incorporate superfoods into your diet that work in the same way as your medications and naturally prevent and control these diseases so that you can reduce the dosage of your medicines as well as the side effects associated with them. This way, your body heals faster than it typically would. Get ready for a healthy tomorrow!

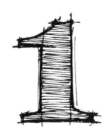

HOW TO USE EAT TO PREVENT AND CONTROL DISEASE COOKBOOK

This cookbook is characterized by

- ✓ Pure vegetarian recipes.
- ✓ Presence of single or multiple superfoods in recipes.
- ✓ Natural sweeteners wherever possible.
- ✓ Healthier versions of the salt like Himalayan pink rock salt, black salt, kala namak mix, and mineral-rich salt mix.
- ✓ Upgraded whole grains mixed flours.
- ✓ Cold-pressed cooking oil.

Cookwares/tools/accessories you need for this cookbook:

- Pressure Cooker
- Hand blender
- Tawa/Skillet
- Muslin cloth
- Steamer
- Convection oven
- Stainless steel kadai/pan
- Mortar and pestle

This cookbook does not use the following ingredients/cooking method/food combinations:

- X Canned foods like canned beans
- X Refined oil
- X Deep frying
- X Salt and milk combination
- X Refined wheat flour
- X Refined white sugar
- X Regular salt
- X No heating of honey

How to steam cook?

You don't need a steamer to steam vegetables and other foods. You can steam them in a large cooker or pot. For this, you need a stainless steel steamer plate/strainer bowl/colander or any perforated plate or bowl that will fit in the cooker or the pot. Keep in mind that it should be kept 2 to 3 inches above the water. You can use a stainless steel pot stand to keep the perforated plate or bowl above the water.

Type of pressure cooker used in this cookbook

This cookbook uses regular pressure cooker with pressure regulator weight valve/whistle.

In this type of pressure cooker, when the steam reaches its peak, it releases steam through the whistle to indicate that the food is cooked. After this, depending on the food, either you have to turn the flame to low and let it cook for some time, or you have to turn off the flame and let all the pressure release naturally. Do not open the lid of the cooker before all the pressure is released. The food continues to cook till all the pressure is released.

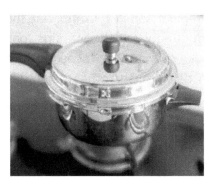

Benefits of using a pressure cooker:

✓ Faster cooking. Saves a lot of time.
✓ Foods retain more nutrition because the steam remains inside and does not escape.
✓ Less messy kitchen.
✓ It can be used as a steamer.

Alternative to pressure cooker: You can cook in a pan covered with a lid, but it will take longer than a pressure cooker.

Healthy Replacements Used in the Cookbook
White Sugar Substitutes

Jaggery, honey, dry fruits, and brown sugar.

White sugar is not used in this cookbook as it provides void calories, which means it has only calories with zero nutrition value. *Eat to Prevent and Control Disease Cookbook* uses jaggery/panela as a sugar substitute because it is the purest form of sugar without any additives and has many health benefits. It is made from sugarcane in an iron vessel, due to which it is an excellent source of iron. If jaggery is not available, you can substitute it with brown sugar. Otherwise, stick to the type of sweetener specified in the recipe for the most authentic flavor.

Jaggery, honey, dried fruits, and brown sugar are healthy alternatives to white sugar. They are nutritious but still are sweet.

Consume them in moderation to get maximum health benefits.

Types of Salt Used in the Cookbook

Himalayan pink rock salt, black salt, kala namak mix, and mineral-rich salt mix.

Mineral-Rich Salt Mix: To upgrade your regular salt, mix Himalayan pink rock salt with your regular salt in 1:1 ratio. Use this mineral-rich salt for better health. Regular salt contains only sodium, whereas Himalayan rock salt is unprocessed and contains traces of iron, magnesium, calcium, and other minerals.

Mineral-rich salt mix is used in all the recipes in this cookbook. Wherever salt is mentioned, it refers to mineral-rich salt mix.

Types of Fat Used in the Cookbook

Mustard oil, extra virgin olive oil, sesame oil, cow ghee, and nuts.

Mustard Oil

Is it banned?
Mustard oil is one of the main cooking oils in many parts of the world, including but not limited to India (particularly North India and West Bengal), Nepal, and Bangladesh. Mustard oil has been used for cooking here for thousands of years, but it is banned in the USA, European Union, and Canada for edible purposes. All commercially available mustard oils in these countries are labeled as *"For external use only."*

The reason for the ban is the presence of erucic acid in mustard oil. Animal studies suggest that high intake of erucic acid is associated with heart diseases. However, this association has not been established for humans as all studies have been done on laboratory animals, and no actual research has been carried on humans. So far, no cases of any harmful effects due to exposure to erucic acid have been reported in humans.

In Indian cooking, mustard oil is used for cooking as well as for dressing. When using mustard oil for cooking, always choose cold-pressed mustard oil instead of refined one to get maximum health benefits.

Substitute of mustard oil

For cooking: Canola oil (but it's refined oil, not pressed oil).

For dressing: Sesame oil or any other cold-pressed oil.

Extra Virgin Olive Oil

To cook or not to cook extra virgin olive oil?

If you cook oil beyond its smoke point, it degrades, and its chemical composition changes. This releases harmful chemicals that get absorbed into the food. It is a myth that extra virgin olive oil can only be used in dressing and not in cooking. The smoke point of extra virgin olive oil is 207 °C. It was believed that extra virgin olive oil oxidizes when cooked due to its low smoke point, but research studies have proven this to be wrong. Everyday cooking doesn't reach 207 °C. Extra virgin olive oil is safe for all types of cooking except for deep frying.

Types of Flour Used in the Cookbook

Whole wheat flour mixed with barley, oats flour made from oats groats, amaranth flour, gram flour, and semolina.

Whole Wheat Barley Mixed Flour

All recipes in this cookbook use whole wheat flour mixed with barley flour. Wherever whole wheat flour is mentioned, it refers to whole wheat flour mixed with barley flour.

Why Barley?

Barley is an excellent source of soluble fiber and antioxidant minerals such as magnesium, copper, selenium, and chromium. Carbohydrates present in barley convert to glucose slowly, without rapidly increasing blood sugar levels. It increases a hormone that helps reduce chronic low-grade inflammation, thus protecting against many chronic diseases as inflammation is the leading cause of cancer, diabetes, arthritis, and many other chronic diseases. If you want to prevent diabetes, then start eating barley regularly.

To make Whole Wheat Barley Mixed Flour: Mix barley flour in the ratio of 1:7 to whole wheat flour. Add 100 grams of barley flour to 700 grams of wheat flour and mix it well. Use this upgraded wheat flour instead of regular wheat flour.

Oat Flour

All recipes in this cookbook use oat flour made from oats groats. Wherever oat flour is mentioned, it refers to oat flour made from oat groats until and unless specified otherwise.

Oat groats are the purest form of oats. It looks similar to whole wheat but is slightly thinner in shape. These are the least processed and highest in nutritional value. The most common type of oats is rolled oats, which have the least nutrition because this variety is the most processed one, and most of the nutrition is lost while processing. They are easy to digest and sometimes fortified (manually added) with essential vitamins and minerals lost during processing, but they are not as healthy and natural as oat groats.

Oat groats are the most nutritious, and even a small intake is enough to provide you with essential nutrients. But they are heavy to digest, so if you eat more, you will feel heaviness in the stomach. So do not eat them too much at a time. Recipes in this cookbook have taken care of the oats amount sufficient for easy digestion and fulfilling nutritional requirements.

If you buy oat groats, once open, consume them within three months. Otherwise, they get spoiled. To grind oats to make oats flour, you need a high-power grinder (above 750 w). Low power mixer grinder will result in coarser flour. You can store oats flour for one month.

For vegan options: Some of the recipes in this cookbook are vegan, but most are vegetarian. You can replace milk and honey with plant-based milk and sweeteners, respectively.

For gluten-free options: Replace wheat, barley, and semolina with any gluten-free flour. The result will be similar without affecting the overall taste of the dish.

Moderation is the key. Even though you are using healthy sugar, salt, or fat types, consuming too much of these can negatively affect your health. They are healthy options but consuming them in excess will nullify their good effects. So consume them in moderation.

Conversions

Degree Celcius to Fahrenheit	Metric Conversion
160 °C = 320 °F	1000 Grams = 1 Kilogram
180 °C = 356 °F	1 Kilogram = 2.2 Pounds
200 °C = 392 °F	1000 Milliliter = 1 Liter
220 °C = 428 °F	28.34 Grams = 1 Ounce

Symbols

Unit	Symbol	Unit	Symbol
Liter	L	Tablespoon	tbsp
Milliliter	ml	Teaspoon	tsp
Gram	g	Degree Celcius	°C
Minute	min	Inch	in

Cup sizes vary from country to country. Therefore, to make it easier to understand, all measurements are given in metric. In general, in this cookbook, 50 grams equals a quarter cup, 100 grams equals a half-cup, and 200 grams equals 1 cup.

Even though cup size varies from country to country, teaspoon and tablespoon sizes are same everywhere. Where quantities are less, the recipes in this cookbook use teaspoons and tablespoons to specify amounts.

1 teaspoon: 5 g | 1 tablespoon: 10 g

In some recipes like masala and mixed dal fry, the ingredients must be mixed in a specific proportion. In these recipes, quantities are given in tablespoons, not metric, to provide accurate ratios.

In general, one tablespoon equals 10 grams, but the actual amount varies according to the ingredients. For example, one tablespoon of coriander seeds contains less than 10 grams. In recipes such as garam masala and panch phoran, where the quantities are specified in teaspoons or tablespoons, they are specified considering their actual weight.

INDIAN COOKING

Eat to Prevent and Control Disease Cookbook's recipes are easy to cook and less time-consuming, you can cook them every day. However, some recipes may take some time to prepare. You can cook them on the weekend when you have a little extra time to invest in cooking. Dishes that are heavy and which keep you full till evening are marked as *weekend special* in the cookbook.

Let's understand a little more about Indian cooking:

Types of Indian Subji

Dry Subji: Dry subji is called *bhujia subji*, which is served as the second subji option in the main course.

Gravy: Gravy subjis are richer and often creamer. These types of subjis are thick and contain nut fats like cashews, melon seeds and peanuts. Gravy subjis taste better when you eat them with raw onions. This is the reason why they are always served with raw onions and lemon. This type of subji is served on special occasions, like when you have visiting guests at your home or when you want to make your Sunday special.

Curry: Curry is called *Rasedar subji*, which is thinner than gravy and has more *Ras* means it contains more water. These are the most common types of subji served in the main course. It may or may not be full of fat. When cooking a rich version on a special occasion, it usually has a high amount of ghee or butter. In this cookbook, you'll find curry-type subjis that don't require high fat and can be eaten guilt-free any day.

The Right Way of Cooking for Enhanced Taste

The right way of cooking gravy

The cooking time is very important while making gravy. In the gravy, the onion-ginger-garlic mixture should be cooked to such an extent that all the rawness of the onion is removed. The nuts should be cooked to a point till the gravy leaves oil. Cook on low or medium-low flame. If you cook on high flame or medium flame, then the mixture will dry quickly, and the gravy will not release oil. If the gravy is not cooked well, then the taste of the gravy will be bland and unbalanced.

The right way of cooking rasedar/curry

Curries/rasedar often do not contain nut fat and are the easiest type of cooking. In this, the spices should be cooked well on low flame for a long time. Once the onions and tomatoes are cooked, add masala and cook on low flame for a long time. It helps to develop the taste. When the masala is cooked well, add water and vegetables to it, bring it to a boil and simmer for 10 minutes on low flame.

The right way to roast nuts/oats

Dry roast while stirring continuously on low flame. Nuts/oats should be roasted until they change color slightly, not until they turn brown or start burning. Turn off the flame and leave them in a pan for 5 minutes. They continue to cook even after turning off the flame in the hot pan.

The right way of roasting whole spices
Roast the whole spices on low flame while stirring continuously until the spices release an aromatic smell.

Tips for enhancing flavor and maximizing health benefits

- To enhance the taste of dry fruits, roast them. It gives a heavenly taste if you roast dry fruits in ghee, whether in as little as half or 1 teaspoon ghee. But it is important to use homemade ghee for roasting as they are rich in flavor and purer than store-bought ghee.

- Soak the beans overnight to reduce the amount of phytic acid, the anti-nutrient of the beans. This helps your body absorb more nutrients from the beans.

- Consumption of beans can cause bloating and flatulence. To avoid such problems, boil the beans thoroughly before using them. Also, add about ¾th to 1 tsp asafoetida while cooking. It helps prevent bloating and flatulence caused by beans.

- If you are using whole spices, then roast them before adding them for better taste. This will enhance their taste.

- Soak the rice in enough water for fifteen minutes before cooking. This shortens the cooking time and lowers the phytic acid content of the rice.

- Preheat the oven to cook evenly. It also reduces the overall cooking time.

Keep Handy!

For Indian cooking, keep the following species ready with you:

Kashmiri red chili powder is characterized by dark red color and is less spicy. This not only gives a bright red color to the food but also keeps the food less spicy.

Fenugreek seeds powder: Dry roast the fenugreek seeds till their color starts changing. Cool them and grind them into a coarse powder.

Coriander powder: Dry roast the whole coriander seeds till they slightly change color. Let them cool down. Grind into a fine powder.

Cumin powder: Dry roast the cumin seeds till they slightly change color. Cool them and grind them finely.

Coriander-cumin powder: For ease, mix coriander powder and cumin powder in ratio of 2:1. Mix 50 g cumin powder with 100 g coriander powder and use this mix instead of coriander powder.

Dry mango powder (*Amchur*): Dry mango powder is made from finely grinding the dry raw mangoes.

Garam masala: This is the most commonly used spice in Indian cooking. Find the recipe in the next chapter.

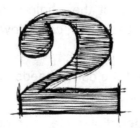

EVERYTHING AT HOME!

Preparation of Indian cuisine requires very few store-bought items. Almost everything can be made at home. Like ghee, curd, and various spices are readily available in the market, but they can be easily made at home. It is an easy and cost-effective method, and once you know the technique, you do not need much expertise.

Here are the add-on recipes necessary to prepare the main dishes of this cookbook. These are either served with meals or are used in cooking to enhance the taste of the food.

MASALA

Masale/spices are an integral part of Indian cooking. These spices have medicinal and therapeutic effects. They help in maintaining the normal functioning of the body. Different spices have different effects on the body. For example, coriander and fennel are good for digestion, while cardamom helps remove toxins from the body. Spices contain flavonoids, a type of antioxidant that helps prevent chronic diseases such as heart disease, diabetes, and cancer.

Spices are warm in nature and produce heat in the body. Eating them in large quantities in winter keeps you warm, while the consumption of spices should be moderate in summer.

The most common masale used in Indian cooking are garam masala, chole masala, and panch phoran. These masale will be used in the recipes of the *Eat to Prevent and Control Disease Cookbook*. These spice blends are readily available in the market, but making them in the home ensures you eat a fresh, flavorsome, and pure form of masala that gives your food the most authentic taste and maximum health benefits.

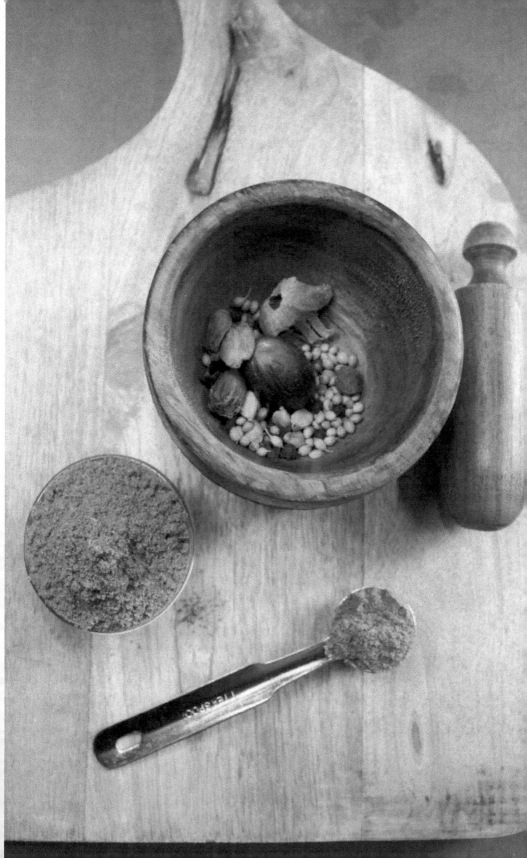

GARAM MASALA

Makes: 70 g | Prep time: 20 mins | Cooking time: 5 mins

Ingredients

Coriander seeds: 3 tbsp	Cumin seeds: 2 tbsp
Black pepper: 1 tbsp	Fennel: 1 tbsp
Dried ginger: 1 inch	Cloves: 8
Black cardamom: 2	Green cardamom: 6
Nutmeg: ½ small	Mace: Half shreds
Bay leaf: 4	Cinnamon stick: 2 inches
Star anise: 1	Carom seeds: ½ tsp
Caraway seeds: ¼ tsp	

Method

1. Dry roast all the ingredients on low flame for 5-7 minutes until your kitchen fills with aromatic spices smell.

2. Turn off the flame. Let the spices cool down.

3. Finely grind the spices. Store garam masala in an airtight container to keep it fresh for longer.

Uses: Almost in all types of food from curry to gravy, from cutlets to dal fry.

Note

It is not that if any of the ingredients are not available, then you cannot make garam masala. If an ingredient is not available, skip it. This will slightly change the taste but is still be better than store-bought garam masala.

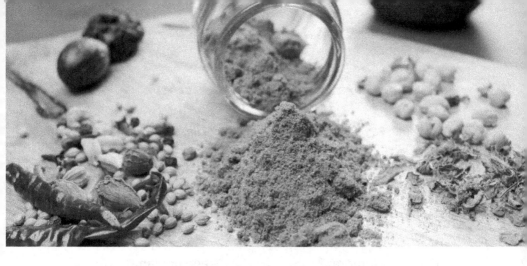

CHOLE MASALA POWDER

Makes: 110 g | Prep time: 15 mins | Cooking time: 5 mins

Ingredients

Coriander seeds: 4 tbsp	Cumin seeds: 2 tbsp
Black pepper: 2 tbsp	Black salt: 1½ tbsp
Dried ginger: 2 inches	Cloves: 10
Black cardamom: 2	Green cardamom: 6
Nutmeg: 1 small	Dry red chilies: 6
Bay leaf: 4 medium or 3 large	Cinnamon: 2 inches
Dried fenugreek leaves: 2 tbsp	Dried mint leaves: 1 tsp
Turmeric powder: 1 tbsp	Dry mango powder: 1½ tbsp

Method

1. Mix turmeric powder, dry mango powder, and black salt.
2. Dry roast the rest of all the ingredients on low flame till spices release an aromatic smell.
3. Grind the roasted spices to a fine powder. Add turmeric powder, dry mango powder, and black salt to it. Mix well. Store in an airtight container.

Uses: Chole masala powder is the main masala used in chole masala and brown chickpeas masala subji.

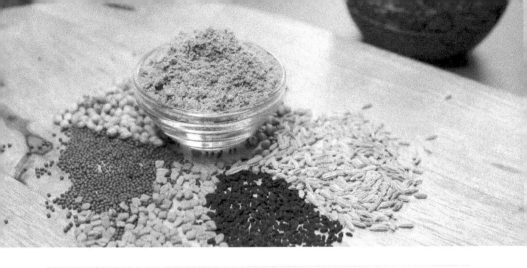

PANCH PHORAN

Makes: 70 g | Prep time: 10 mins | Cooking time: 5 mins

Ingredients

Coriander seeds: 4 tbsp	Fennel seeds: 2 tbsp
Fenugreek seeds: 1 tbsp	Whole dry red chilies: 2
Nigella seeds: 1 tsp	Mustard seeds: 1 tsp

Method

1. Remove the stem from chilies. If you want to make the chilies less spicy, remove the seeds.

2. Dry roast all ingredients except mustard seeds till the spices release an aromatic smell.

3. Cool the spices. Add mustard seeds and grind them finely.

4. Store Panch Phoran in an airtight container.

Uses: Panch phoran is used in stuffed vegetables such as stuffed bell pepper, stuffed bitter gourd, and stuffed pointed gourd.

KALA NAMAK MIX

Makes: 440 g | Prep time: 20 mins

Ingredients

Black salt: 200 g	Rock salt: 100 g
Roasted cumin seeds: 50 g	Roasted carom seeds: 50 g
Black pepper: 25 g	Asafoetida: 5 g
Clove: 10	Green cardamom: 5

Method

1. Dry roast cumin seeds and carom seeds.

2. If you are using whole black salt and rock salt, then crush black salt and rock salt with the help of a pestle.

3. Grind cumin, carom seeds, black pepper, cloves, cardamom, and asafoetida together.

4. Add black salt and rock salt and grind again into fine powder.

5. Store in an airtight container for up to two months. Do not open the lid frequently to keep the kala namak mix fresh.

6. Fill the Kala Namak Mix in a small salt sprinkler for daily use.

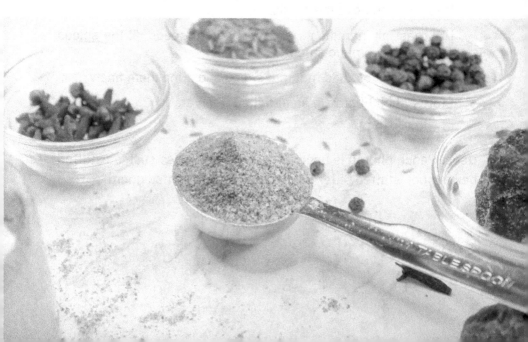

MILK PRODUCTS

DESI GHEE

There is not only one way to make ghee at home. Ghee can be made from malai (cream top of milk), butter, and curd. Using cow's milk to make ghee is a great way to boost your health. Cow's milk ghee has a high smoke point, making it safe for cooking that requires high temperatures, such as deep-frying. Including ghee in your diet is beneficial when you replace other forms of fat with ghee, not when you take ghee as an additional source of fat. To get the complete nutrition of ghee, replace butter, margarine with ghee.

Makes: 125 ml | Prep time: 7-10 days | Cooking time: 45 mins

Ingredients

Cream top of cow's milk: 500 g

Method

1. Boil 2 liters of milk. Turn off the flame. Let it cool down completely.
2. After 4-5 hours, you will see a thick layer of cream (*malai*) on

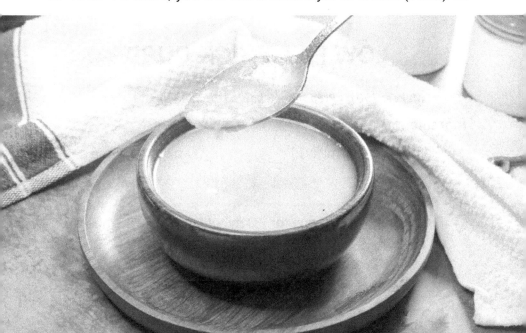

the top of the milk. Collect this cream and store it in an airtight container in the freezer.

3. Repeat this every day till you collect 500 g of cream. It will take around 7 to 10 days. Days may vary due to the quality and quantity of milk. Be sure to keep it in the freezer in an airtight container.

4. To make ghee, take it out from the freezer and leave it for 3-4 hours till it comes to room temperature. Now using a hand blender, blend the cream so that it becomes smooth and uniform.

5. Take a pan and pour smooth cream into it. Bring it to a boil and let it boil for about half an hour till the transparent ghee starts separating.

6. Let it boil for another 15 to 20 minutes till the ghee separates completely and the milk solids turn brown. Stir continuously.

7. Turn off the flame. Leave for 15 minutes. Strain the ghee, discard the solid brown part and collect the ghee in a container. Use as required.

Tip

Usually, the cream is whipped until butter and buttermilk separate, and butter is used to make ghee, but this results in yellowish thin ghee. To make granular ghee, it is necessary to blend the cream until it is smooth and uniform, not until butter starts separating.

LOW FAT THICK CURD

Makes: 750 g | Prep time: 8 hours | Cooking time: 10 mins

Ingredients

Skimmed cow's milk: 1 L	Curd starter: 1 tsp

Method

1. Blend curd with a spoon for 2-3 minutes to make it smooth.

2. Boil the milk for 10 minutes. Let the milk cool down. To make perfect thick curd, keep the milk lukewarm, neither completely cold nor too hot. Add curd in lukewarm milk and mix well.

3. Cover with a lid and keep it in a warm and dry place overnight. To make it even more fat-free, remove the layer of cream from the top of the curd the following day.

4. If you need the curd on the same day, pre-heat the oven at 160 °C for 5 to 10 minutes. Switch off the oven. Put the covered curd in the hot oven for 3-4 hours. Your low-fat curd is ready.

Hung curd

1. Put the curd in a muslin cloth and tie it. Squeeze to remove excess water. Hang it on a tap or any other place for 5-6 hours.

2. Take out the hung curd in a bowl. Blend with a spoon for 2 minutes. Your creamy hung curd is ready.

Tips

1. Curd starter is nothing but leftover curd from the previous batch of curd making. If you are making curd for the first time at home, you can buy a curd starter from a dairy shop, or any other store-bought curd will work as well. For next batch, use a teaspoon of the curd you made as curd starter.

2. Do not add too much curd starter to the milk. The more curd starter you add, the more sour your curd will be.

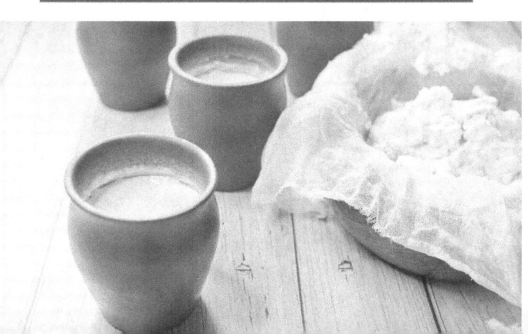

CHUTNEY

Chutneys are the dip used with an evening snack, paratha, or added to a dish to enhance the taste.

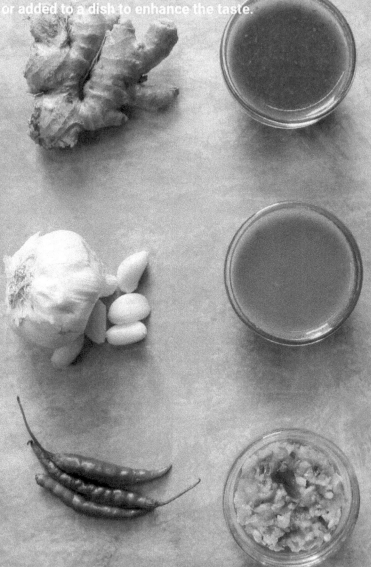

GREEN CHUTNEY

Makes: 200 ml | Prep time: 15 mins

Ingredients

Coriander leaves: 100 g	Ginger: ½ inch
Garlic/Green garlic: 25 g	Green chilies: 4
Salt: To taste	Dry mango powder: ½ tsp
Water: 75 ml	

Method

1. Grind all the ingredients except salt in 25 ml water.
2. Add salt and the rest of the water. Mix well.
3. Store in an airtight container in the refrigerator for up to 2 weeks.

RED GARLIC CHUTNEY

Makes: 60 ml | Prep time: 10 mins

Ingredients

Garlic: 15 cloves	Red chili powder: 1 tbsp
Water: 50 ml	Salt: To taste

Method

1. Grind all the ingredients together except salt.
2. Add salt and store in the refrigerator for up to 5 days.

KHUNUA

Makes: 20 g | Prep time: 15 mins

Ingredients

Garlic: 15-20 cloves	Mustard oil: 1 tsp
Salt: To taste	Green chilies: 3

Method

1. Crush garlic and chilies in a mortar using the pestle.
2. Fill it in an airtight container. Add salt and mustard oil and mix well. Store in the refrigerator for up to 5 days.

3

EAT TO
BOOST
IMMUNITY

As we have covered the immunity-boosting superfoods in detail in *Eat to Prevent and Control Disease*, we will now see how you can incorporate those superfoods into your diet in this cookbook.

This chapter focuses on foods that boost immunity as well as superfoods that have therapeutic and medicinal effects on the body. The superfoods on which the recipes of this chapter are based are:

- **Green tea**.
- Herbs that have therapeutic effects: **Turmeric, fenugreek seeds,** and **basil leaves**.
- Nutrient-dense vegetables and legumes: **Sweet potato** and **mung sprouts**.
- Vitamin C-rich foods: **Red** and **green bell pepper**.
- Foods rich in vitamin A: **Sweet potato**.
- Omega-3 fats and zinc-rich foods: **Cashew nuts, almonds, walnuts, flax seeds, etc**.

THE ULTIMATE GREEN TEA KADHA

Taking kadha every day supports immune system and protects against the common cold, viral infections, and flu. Start your day with the ultimate green tea kadha and see how less you get sick.

Serves: 4 | Prep time: 5 mins | Cooking time: 10 mins | Beverage

Ingredients

Green tea: 4 tsp	Fresh turmeric: 1½ inches
Carom seeds: 1 tsp	Fresh ginger: 1½ inches
Cloves: 6	Cinnamon: ½ inch
Bay leaf: 1	Basil leaves: 10
Black pepper: 6	Water: 900 ml

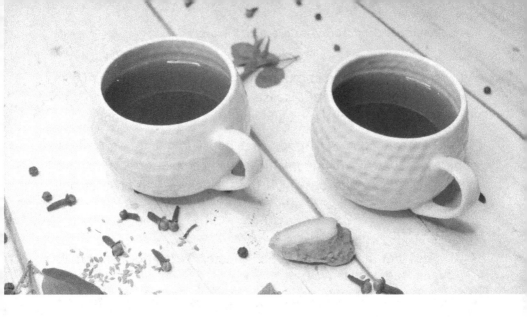

Method

1. Take all the ingredients except green tea and water in a mortar and crush them using a pestle. Put the herbs in a pan and add water.

2. Bring the kadha to a boil. Simmer for 5 minutes on medium flame.

3. Add green tea and simmer for another 5-8 minutes or till the kadha reduces to 600 ml. Turn off the flame. Strain kadha and drink hot.

Tip

If you want to make the kadha sweet, then add jaggery while simmering. If you have a cold, sore throat, or cough, take the kadha three times a day, do not add any sweet, and increase the quantity of black pepper to 10. Take a sip, tighten your lips and exhale through your nose. This will help in relieving nasal congestion.

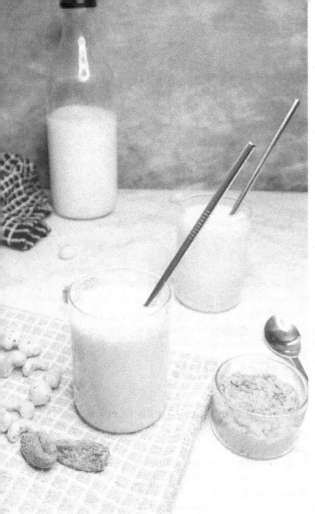

DRY FRUITS MILK

Serves: 4 | Prep time: 5 mins | Cooking time: 20 mins | Beverage

Ingredients

Dried coconut: 50 g	Poppy seeds: 10 g
Dried date: 50 g	Almonds: 50 g
Cashew nuts: 50 g	Walnuts: 30 g
Pumpkin seed: 20 g	Fox nuts: 20 g
Water: 150 ml	Ghee: ½ tsp
Milk: 1.5 L	

Method

1. Soak all dry fruits in water overnight. Soak poppy seeds separately. Next day, rinse the dry fruits with fresh water.

2. Remove seeds from dried dates. Grind all the ingredients together with 150 ml of water.

3. Heat ghee in a pan. Add dry fruits paste to it. Cook for 5 to 10 minutes or until all water is evaporated. It will look like halwa at this stage. Turn off the flame. You can also eat it as halwa.

4. Boil milk in a separate saucepan. Add dry fruits halwa in milk as required. Mix well. Simmer for 5 minutes.

5. Cool the Dry Fruits Milk. Stir with a spoon and serve hot.

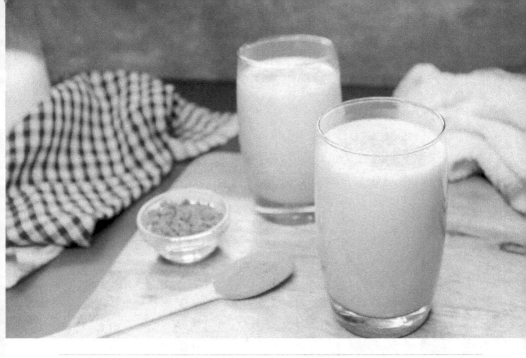

GOLDEN MILK

Serves: 4 | Prep time: 5 mins | Cooking time: 10 mins | Beverage

Ingredients

Fresh turmeric: 2 inches or Turmeric powder: 1 tbsp	Milk: 1 L

Method

1. Boil the milk. Peel the fresh turmeric and crush it in a mortar with the help of a pestle.

2. Add crushed fresh turmeric to the milk. Simmer for 5 minutes. Turn off the flame. Strain the milk. Let it cool down.

3. Drink it just before bed while the golden milk is still hot.

Tip

Use fresh turmeric in the winter season and turmeric powder in other seasons when fresh turmeric is not available.

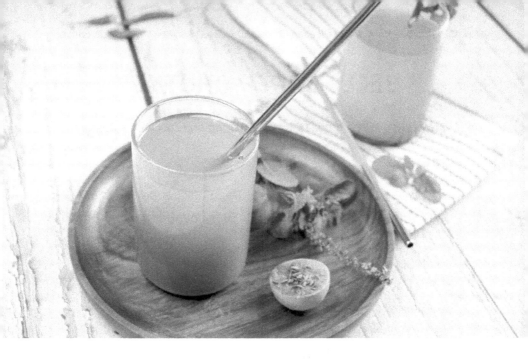

TULSI SUMMER DRINK

Serves: 4 | Prep time: 15 mins | Beverage

Ingredients

Indian Tulsi/Basil leaves: 50   Ginger: 2 inches
Green chilies: 2   Cumin seeds: 1 tbsp
Lemon: 2 tbsp   Chilled water: 1 L
Kala namak mix: To taste

Method

1. Roast cumin seeds till they slightly change color.
2. Take basil leaves, ginger, chilies, and roasted cumin seeds in a grinder jar. Grind with about 50 ml water to a fine paste.
3. Pass the paste through a strainer. Discard the solid part.
4. Add the remaining water, kala namak mix, and lemon juice.
5. Chill tulsi summer drink in the refrigerator for 2 hours.
6. Enjoy the tangy Tulsi Summer Drink on a hot afternoon.

BELL PEPPER CHUTNEY

Makes: 200 g | Prep time: 15 mins | Cooking time: 25 mins | Condiment

Ingredients

Red bell pepper: 1 large/160 g	Green bell pepper: 1 small/50 g
Apple cider vinegar: 1 tbsp	Black pepper powder: ½ tsp
Jaggery: 20 g	Cloves: 6
Chopped onion: 1 large	Chopped ginger: 1 tbsp
Chopped garlic: 2 tbsp	Bay leaf: 1
Kashmiri red chili powder: 1 tbsp	Salt: To taste
Sesame oil: 1½ tbsp	Water: 200 ml

Method

1. Place a metal rack over a stove-top burner over direct flame. Put red and green bell pepper on the metal rack and roast on low flame.

2. Rotate and roast the bell peppers from all sides. It will take around 10-15 minutes. Take them off the flame.

3. Take bell peppers in a bowl and pour 100 ml hot water over them. Cover with a lid and keep aside for 15 minutes.

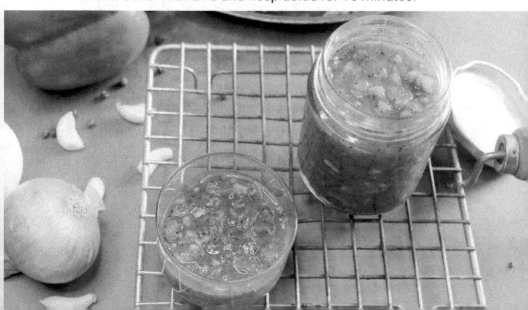

4. Blend bell peppers with water to a smooth paste. Keep aside.

5. Heat oil in a pan. Add bay leaf, cloves, ginger, and garlic. Cook on medium flame till they start turning brown.

6. Add chopped onions and cook for 6-8 minutes.

7. Add Kashmiri red chili powder and cook for 30 seconds.

8. Add bell pepper paste. Mix well and cook for 5 minutes.

9. Add salt, black pepper powder, jaggery, and apple cider vinegar. Mix well.

10. Add 100 ml water. Cover the chutney with a lid and cook for 10 minutes on low flame. Stir occasionally.

11. When oil appears on the top of the chutney, it means that the chutney is ready. Turn off the flame and let the chutney cool down.

12. Fill it in an airtight glass container and store it in the refrigerator for up to 2 weeks.

13. Serve the Bell Pepper Chutney with cutlet or as a dip or spread over bread and chapati or use in veg rolls.

METHI PYAZ PARATHA

Serves: 4 | Prep time: 30 mins Cooking time: 20 mins | Breakfast

Ingredients

Whole wheat flour: 400 g	Sprouted fenugreek seeds: 40 g
Onion: 4 ½ medium	Carom seeds: 1 tsp
Nigella seeds: ½ tsp	Green chilies: 2
Roasted cumin seeds: 1 tsp	Salt: To taste
Coriander leaves: 20 g	Asafoetida: ¼ tsp
Extra virgin olive oil: 2 tbsp	Water: 100 ml

Method

1. Grind sprouted fenugreek seeds with 100 ml water.

2. Dry roast cumin seeds. Crush them in a mortar with a pestle.

3. Finely chop onion and green chilies.

4. Take all ingredients in a bowl except oil and knead to make a stiff dough without adding any additional water. If it seems too dry, add 2 tbsp of water. Make sure not to add too much water as the onion will release water later. Cover and rest the dough for 15 minutes.

5. Take one dough ball, dip it in the dry whole wheat flour, and dust off the excess flour. Use a rolling pin to roll the dough into a circle.

6. Heat the pan/griddle/skillet (Tawa) on medium-high flame. Place the paratha on the tawa. Cook for about a minute or until the paratha starts puffing from the base in some places.

7. Flip the paratha and spread 3-4 drops of olive oil. Cook for 2 minutes until lightly browned.

8. Flip the paratha again and pour 3-4 drops of olive oil on top, and spread it evenly over the surface. Press the paratha gently with a flat spatula so that the paratha gets cooked evenly.

9. Once brown spots appear on both sides of the paratha, take it out on a serving plate. Similarly, make all the parathas.

10. Enjoy Methi Pyaz Paratha with red chutney, green chutney, and curd.

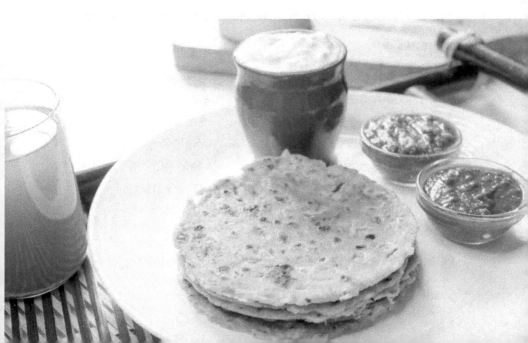

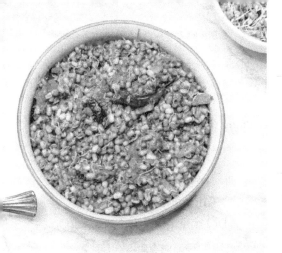

SPROUTED MUNG BEAN SUBJI

Serves: 4 | Prep time: 15 mins | Cooking time: 30 mins | Side dish

Ingredients

Sprouted mung beans: 250 g	Onion: 2 medium
Tomato: 2 medium	Ginger: 1 inch
Garlic: 6 cloves	Whole red chilies: 2
Mustard seeds: 1 tsp	Cumin seeds: ½ tsp
Coriander-cumin powder: 1½ tsp	Garam masala: ½ tsp
Jaggery: 15 g	Asafoetida: ½ tsp
Bay leaf: 1	Turmeric powder: ½ tsp
Water: 350 ml	Oil: 1 tbsp
Salt: To taste	

Method

1. Heat oil in a pan. Add asafoetida, bay leaf, red chilies, mustard seeds, and cumin seeds. Cook till seeds start crackling.

2. Add ginger and garlic. Cook for 2 minutes. Add chopped onions. Cook on low flame for 5-7 minutes.

3. Add turmeric powder, garam masala, coriander-cumin powder. Mix well. Cover and cook for 5 minutes on low flame.

4. Add chopped tomatoes and salt. Cook for 5 minutes.

5. Add sprouted mung beans and jaggery. Mix well and cook for 5 minutes. Add water.

6. Cover and cook for 10 minutes on low flame. Serve hot.

STUFFED BELL PEPPER

Serves: 4 | Prep time: 15 mins | Cooking time: 40 mins | Main course

Ingredients

Green bell pepper: 4 large	Sweet potato: 600 g
Red chili powder: ½ tsp	Chopped ginger: 1 tsp
Chopped garlic: 1 tbsp	Dry mango powder: ½ tsp
Cumin seeds: ½ tsp	Asafoetida: ¼ tsp
Panch phoran: 1½ tsp	Salt: To taste

Method

1. Steam the sweet potatoes. Remove the skin and mash them.

2. Heat oil in a pan. Add asafoetida and cumin seeds. When cumin seeds start turning brown, add ginger and garlic. Cook for 2 minutes. Add mashed sweet potatoes. Mix well and cook for 5 minutes.

3. Add salt, dry mango powder, red chili powder, and panch phoran masala. Mix well. Cook for 10 minutes on medium flame. Stir occasionally. Turn off the flame and let the stuffing cool down.

4. Wash the bell peppers and remove the top portion and seeds. Stuff the sweet potato mixture in each bell pepper. Brush each bell pepper with oil. Sprinkle salt over each bell pepper.

5. Place the stuffed bell peppers in a metal rack and bake in a pre-heated oven at 180 °C for 15 minutes. Flip the bell peppers and bake again for another 10-15 minutes. Serve hot.

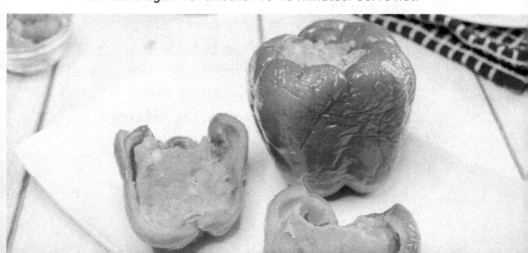

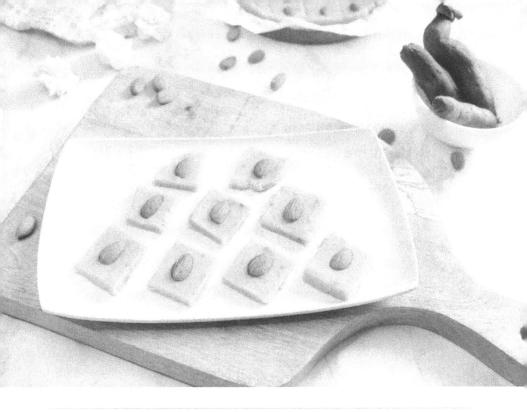

SWEET POTATO BURFI

Serves: 4 | Prep time: 20 mins | Cooking time: 40 mins | Dessert

Ingredients

Sweet potato: 300 g (purple variety)

Jaggery: 60-70 g

Water: 100 ml

Ghee: 1 tbsp

Almond: 10 -15

Method

1. Steam cook sweet potatoes. Remove skin and mash them using a potato masher or spoon.

2. Put jaggery in a pan. Heat it on low flame. When it starts melting, add water to it.

3. Turn the flame to medium and let the mix boil till *one string chashni* is formed. To check, put a drop of jaggery chashni on

a plate. Let it cool down for 15 seconds. Take it between your thumb and index finger and check if it forms a string while separating your fingers. If it forms a string, it means it is done. If not, cook for another minute and check again.

4. Turn the flame to low and add mashed sweet potatoes and mix well. Keep stirring it continuously so that it does not stick to the bottom. Once mixed well, cook it on low to medium flame.

5. It will start forming a ball. At this stage, add 1 tbsp of ghee. Mix well till it stops sticking to the bottom and forms a non-sticky ball.

6. Turn off the flame and let it cool down a bit.

7. Take it out on the greased work platform and knead it for 5 minutes to make the smooth burfi.

8. Put butter paper on a flat plate and spread the dough on it. Roll it by pressing with palm or roll it with the help of a rolling pin. Keep the thickness from 0.5 cm to 0.75 cm. Let it cool down.

9. Dry roast 10-15 almonds and open them in the vertical half.

10. Grease your palm with about ¼ tsp ghee and pat the top of the burfi. Cut in squares and stick half an almond on each piece. Keep in refrigerator and consume within 2 days.

Tips

1. Make sure to steam sweet potatoes; do not boil them. Boiling makes sweet potato mushy and strong-flavored that disrupts the balanced taste of burfi.

2. The quantity of jaggery depends on the sweetness of the sweet potato. So adjust the jaggery quantity accordingly.

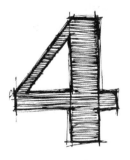

EAT FOR MAXIMUM HEALTH BENEFITS

(THE ULTIMATE NUTRIENT COMBINATIONS)

Nutrients need to be adequately absorbed into the body to provide health benefits. Some nutrients are rapidly eliminated from your body without being absorbed, and you don't get their health benefits. Various factors affect the absorption of nutrients. Foods require a favorable environment and the presence of specific vitamins and minerals inside the body to be absorbed. If the foods aren't absorbed into your body, you don't get the health benefits. Fortunately, you can increase the absorption of food by combining it with other foods that provide the necessary environment for their absorption and inhibit their metabolism. As a result, nutrients are more available to be absorbed into the bloodstream, and you get maximum health benefits from them.

Here are recipes of nutrient combinations that provide maximum health benefits when eaten together:

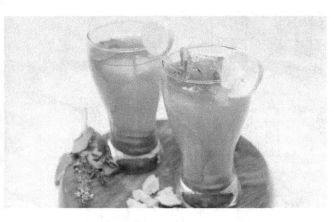

GINGER GREEN ICED TEA

Green tea + Lemon

Serves: 4 | Prep time: 20 mins | Cooking time: 10 mins | Beverage

Ingredients

Green tea: 4 tsp/ 4 green tea bag	Basil leaves: 20
Mint leaves: 20	Ginger: 2 inches
Lemon: 2 tbsp	Water: 1 L
Ice cubes: 12 (optional)	Lemon slices: For garnish
Honey: To taste (optional)	

Method

1. Crush ginger with a pestle. Add green tea, basil leaves, and ginger to the water. Bring it to a boil. Simmer for 5-7 minutes.

2. Add mint leaves and lemon juice and turn off the flame. Cover and leave for 15 minutes till tea reaches room temperature.

3. Strain the tea. Add honey if you want to sweeten your tea. Chill the tea in the refrigerator for 3-4 hours.

4. Pour the chilled ginger green iced tea into glasses. Add lemon slices, basil leaves, and ice cubes. Enjoy this summer drink.

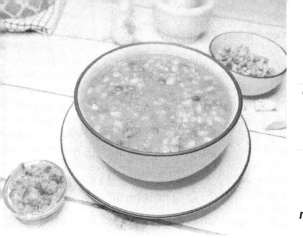

7 ANAJ WITH KHUNUA

Phytic acid + Water

Serves: 4 | Prep time: 10 mins | Cooking time: 15 mins Breakfast

Ingredients

Brown chickpeas: 50 g	Whole yellow peas: 50 g
Whole wheat: 80 g	Whole pigeon peas: 50 g
Whole mung beans: 50 g	Soybean: 50 g
Peanuts: 50 g	Water: 850 ml
Khunua: 1 tsp/as required	Mustard oil: 1 tsp
Salt: To taste	

Method

1. Soak all 7 anaj overnight in enough water. Next morning wash all anaj with fresh water 4 to 5 times.

2. Put all 7 anaj in the pressure cooker. Add water and ½ tsp salt only as khunua already contains salt. Pressure cook for 5-7 whistles. Open the lid. Add khunua and mustard oil. Mix well.

3. Start your day with the soupy 7 Anaj with the heavenly taste of raw garlic and mustard oil.

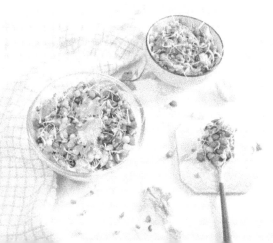

MIXED SPROUTS

Vitamin C + Iron | Complete protein

Serves: 4 | Prep time: 15 mins | Breakfast/Snack

Ingredients

Sprouted brown chickpeas: 75 g	Sprouted mung beans: 75 g
Sprouted horse gram: 50 g	Boiled corn kernels: 50 g
Sprouted fenugreek seeds: 20 g	Sprouted peanuts: 25 g
Apple: 2	Cucumber: 1
Pomegranate: 1	Tomato: 1
Onion: 1	Chopped green chilies: To taste
Lemon juice: 1 tbsp	Kala namak mix: To taste
Chopped mint leaves: 1 tbsp	Coriander leaves: 1 tbsp

Method

1. Chop apple, cucumber, chilies, onion, and tomato.
2. Put all the ingredients of mixed sprouts in a bowl. Mix well.
3. Leave for 10 minutes. Enjoy fresh mixed sprouts.

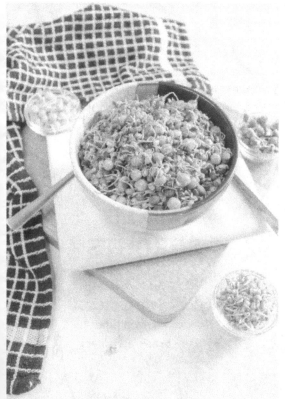

EASY-TO-DIGEST SPROUTS

Serves: 4 | Prep time: 5 mins | Cooking time: 10 mins | Breakfast

Ingredients

Sprouted brown chickpeas: 75 g	Sprouted whole pigeon peas: 50 g
Sprouted mung beans: 75 g	Sprouted horse: gram: 50 g

Black pepper powder: ¼ tsp	Ginger: 2 inches
Asafoetida: ¼ tsp	Salt: To taste
Water: 75 ml	Mustard oil: 1 tsp

Method

1. Heat oil in a pressure cooker. Add asafoetida, chopped green chilies, and cumin seeds. When cumin seeds start changing color, add all sprouts.

2. Cook for 5 minutes. Add black pepper powder, salt, and water.

3. Pressure cook for 2-3 whistles. Turn off the flame. Let the pressure release naturally. Enjoy the Easy-to-Digest Sprouts every morning.

FRUIT CHAAT

Vitamin D + Calcium | Folate + Vitamin B12

Serves: 4 | Prep time: 20 mins | Snack

Ingredients

Thick curd: 250 g	Apple: 2
Banana: 2	Pomegranate: 1
Orange: 1	Papaya: 50 g
Kiwi: 2	Musk melon: 50 g
Plus, any seasonal fruits	Almond: 10

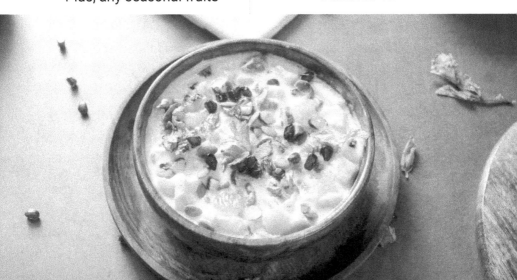

Pistachios: 10	Walnut: 3 kernels
Pumpkin seeds: 3 tsp	Cumin seeds: 1 tsp
Chopped mint leaves: 2 tbsp	Honey: 1 tbsp
Kala namak mix: To taste	Dry mango powder: ¼ tsp

Method

1. Dry roast cumin seeds for 2 minutes and coarsely grind them.
2. Smoothen the curd by blending it with a spoon for 2 minutes.
3. Chop all the ingredients. Add them in curd. Mix well.
4. Add cumin seeds, dry mango powder, kala namak mix, and honey to it. Mix well. Refrigerate for 1 hour. Serve chilled.

MUSHROOM IN CREAMY SPINACH GRAVY

Vitamin C + Iron Vitamin D + Calcium Folate + Vitamin B12

Servess: 4 | Prep time: 15 mins | Cooking time: 1 hour | Main course (Weekend Special)

Ingredients

Button mushrooms: 200 g	Spinach: 200 g
Cashew nuts: 30	Melon seeds: 20 g
Onion: 4 medium	Tomato: 3 medium
Ginger: 1 ½ inch	Garlic: 10 cloves
Turmeric powder: ¼ tsp	Garam masala powder: 1 tsp
Coriander powder: ½ tsp	Red chili powder: ½ tsp
Asafoetida: ¼ tsp	Bay leaf: 1
Cumin seeds: ½ tsp	Water: 250 ml
Lemon juice: 1 tsp	Salt: To taste
Ghee: 2 tbsp	

For Tadka

Chopped garlic: 1 tbsp　　　Kashmiri red chili powder: ½ tsp

Asafoetida: ¼ tsp　　　　　　Ghee: 1 tsp

Method

1. Wash spinach thoroughly. Discard the stems and use fresh spinach leaves only. Blanch the spinach in 100 ml of water with salt and lemon juice for 1 minute. Let it cool and blend to a smooth paste.

2. Soak cashew nuts and melon seeds in 100 ml of hot water for 15 minutes. Grind to a fine white paste.

3. Grind together onion, ginger, and garlic to a fine paste. Separately blend tomatoes without adding water.

4. Cut mushroom into 1-inch cubes. Heat ½ tsp of ghee. Add mushroom pieces and sauté for 10 minutes.

5. Heat ghee in another pan. Add asafoetida, bay leaf, and cumin seeds. When cumin seeds start changing color, add the onion-ginger-garlic paste. Cover and cook on low flame for 10 minutes till the raw taste of onion goes away completely.

6. Add tomato paste and salt. Mix well. Cover and cook for 5 minutes. Add turmeric powder, garam masala, coriander powder, and red chili powder. Cover and cook on low flame for

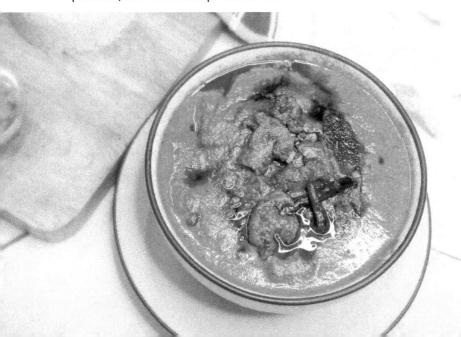

10 minutes. Stir occasionally.

7. Add cashew-melon paste. Cover and cook on low flame for 15 minutes till the gravy leaves oil.

8. Add spinach paste and mix well. Bring it to a boil. If the gravy is too thick, add 50 to 100 ml water. Simmer for 5 minutes on low flame.

9. Add mushrooms. Mix and simmer for 2 minutes. Turn off the flame.

For Tadka

1. Add asafoetida, chopped garlic, and red chili powder to the hot ghee. Cook for 2-3 minutes.

2. Add tadka to mushroom in creamy spinach gravy. Cover and leave for 5 minutes. Serve with chapati and rice

WINTER CURRY

Turmeric + Black pepper

Serves: 4 | Prep time: 20 mins | Cooking time: 1 hour | Main course

Ingredients

Cauliflower: 250 g	Sweet potato: 100 g
Carrot: 100 g	Garlic: 8-10 cloves
Ginger: 2 inches	Onion: 3 medium
Tomato: 2 medium	Green chilies: 2
Turmeric powder: ½ tsp	Black pepper powder: ¼ tsp
Garam masala: 1 tsp	Coriander-cumin powder: 1 tsp
Red chili powder: ¼ tsp	Asafoetida: ½ tsp
Bay leaf: 1	Cumin seeds: ½ tsp
Fenugreek seeds powder: ¼ tsp	Salt: To taste
Mustard oil: 2½ tbsp	Water: 300 ml

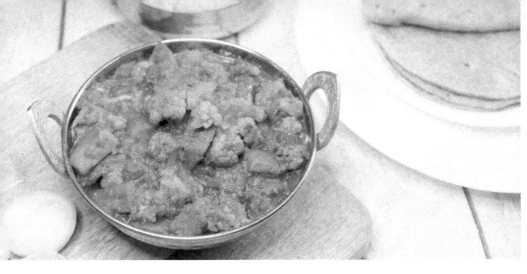

Method

1. Peel sweet potato and carrot. Cut cauliflower, sweet potato, and carrot into one-inch cubes.

2. Grind together onion, ginger, garlic, and green chilies coarsely. Make sure not to make a fine paste. Grind tomatoes separately.

3. Heat 1 tsp of oil in a pan. Add asafoetida and cauliflower. Cook on low flame for 10 minutes till brown spots appear on the cauliflower. Take out the cauliflower from the pan.

4. In the same pan, add ½ tsp oil. Add sweet potato pieces. Cook for 10 minutes until they slightly turn brown. Remove them from heat. Add ½ tsp oil and add carrot. Cook for 7-10 minutes. Remove them from heat.

5. Heat 1½ tbsp oil in the same pan. Add asafoetida, bay leaf, cumin seeds, and fenugreek seeds powder. Cook for 2 minutes. Add onion-ginger-garlic paste. Cook for 10 minutes.

6. Add turmeric, black pepper powder, red chili powder, garam masala, coriander-cumin powder. Cook for 5 minutes on low flame. Add tomato paste. Mix well. Cook for 5-7 minutes.

7. Add salt and 300 ml water. Add cauliflower, carrot, and sweet potato pieces. If you prefer more *ras*, add 50 ml-100 ml more water as per your taste. Do not add too much water as it will dilute the flavor.

8. Cover with a lid and cook on low flame for 10 minutes. Turn off the flame. Serve with chapati and rice.

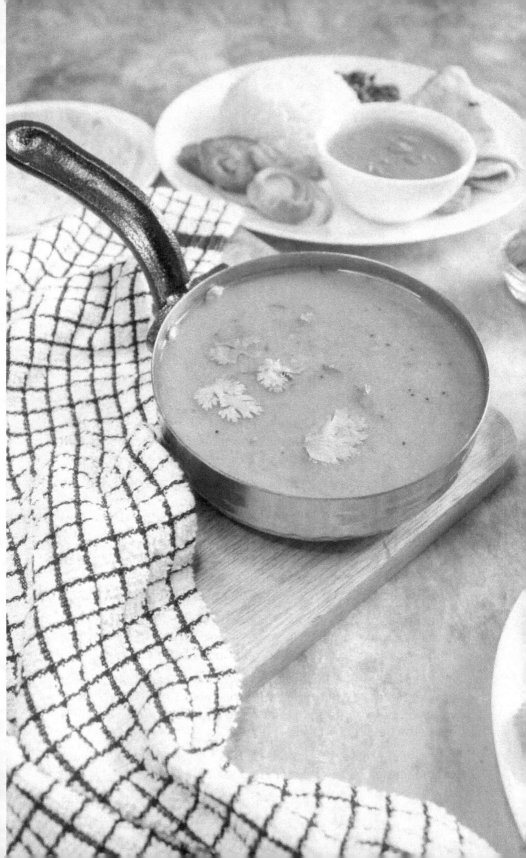

MASALA MIXED DAL

Vitamin C + Iron | Tomato + Olive oil | Phytic acid + Water

Serves: 4 | Prep time: 15 mins | Cooking: 30 mins | Main course

Ingredients

Split yellow pigeon pea: 4 tbsp	Split green pigeon pea: 2 tbsp
Red lentils: 2 tbsp	Split yellow mung beans: 2 tbsp
Tomato: 1 medium	Salt: To taste
Asafoetida: ½ tsp	Peanuts: 2 tbsp
Turmeric powder: 1 tsp	Coriander powder: ½ tsp
Garam masala: 1 tsp	Cumin seeds: ½ tsp
Mustard seeds: 1 tsp	Dried red chilies: 2
Curry leaves: 5-6	Water: 700 ml
Kokum: 3	Olive oil: 1 tbsp

Method

1. Soak peanuts in hot water for 15 minutes. Soak kokum in about 100 ml of hot water for 15 minutes.

2. Wash lentils with fresh water and soak in enough water for 15 minutes to reduce cooking time and to remove phytic acid.

3. Discard the water. Take split yellow pigeon pea, split green pigeon pea, red lentils, split yellow moong beans, salt, turmeric powder, asafoetida, and chopped tomatoes in a pressure cooker. Add 400 ml of water and pressure cook for 4 whistles. The dal should be mushy. Blend smooth with a hand blender.

4. Heat oil in a pan. Add asafoetida, red chilies, mustard seeds, and cumin seeds. When seeds start crackling, add curry leaves. Add dal mix, soaked peanuts, and rest of the water.

5. Let the dal boil. Add salt, garam masala, coriander powder, and kokum along with water (in which it was soaked).

6. Cook the dal on a medium flame for 10 minutes. Turn off the flame. Garnish with coriander leaves.

Kokum substitute: If kokum is unavailable, you can add 1 tbsp of lemon juice (after turning off the flame, not while cooking).

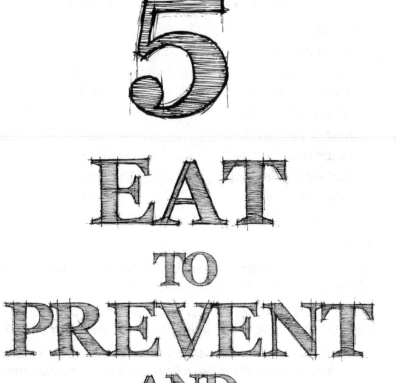

5

EAT
TO
PREVENT
AND
CONTROL
DIABETES

Diabetes is a chronic disease in which the body either does not produce insulin or does not use insulin effectively, resulting in high blood sugar levels.

Healthy diet plays an important role in preventing and managing diabetes. Controlling diabetes isn't just about avoiding foods that can increase your blood sugar levels. It is also about choosing the right foods which naturally prevent and control diabetes.

Healthy Alternatives to Prevent and Control Diabetes:

Replace Potatoes with Sweet Potatoes

Sweet potatoes have a sweeter taste than potatoes and give the false impression that they increase sugar levels much faster than potatoes. But this is not true. The glycemic index of sweet potatoes is lower than that of potatoes. This is because the carbohydrates present in sweet potatoes are different than in potatoes. Carbohydrates in potatoes are quickly broken down and converted into sugar, causing a sudden spike in blood sugar levels.

On the other hand, the carbohydrates present in sweet potatoes slowly convert to sugar. So, sugar releases into the blood slowly and does not cause a sudden spike in blood sugar levels. This makes sweet potatoes safe for diabetic people when consumed in moderation.

Replace Sugar with Dry Fruits

Using dry fruits in place of sugar is a healthy option for people with diabetes. Dried fruits are rich in fiber, antioxidants, and healthy monounsaturated fats. When consumed in moderation, dried fruits such as dates (2–3 a day), raisins (2 tbsp a day), and figs can be safely used to sweeten desserts. However, each person may be in a different stage of diabetes. Depending on your diabetic condition, your doctor can tell you exactly how many dried fruits you should eat in a day, so consult your doctor to find out the right amount for you. Dried fruits are being used as a substitute for sugar in the following recipes. If it is not suitable for you, replace it with artificial sweetener or do as suggested by your doctor.

The recipes in this chapter are based on superfoods that have therapeutic effects and help prevent and control diabetes through the following mechanism of actions:

- Foods that mimick the action of insulin: **Bitter gourd**.
- Foods that increase glucose-induced insulin release: **Fenugreek**.
- Foods that are high in dietary fiber: **Bottle gourd** and **fenugreek**.
- Foods that reduce the risk of insulin resistance: **Bottle gourd, chickpeas,** and **green peas**.
- Foods that increase glucose metabolism and enhance insulin sensitivity: **Bottle gourd, bitter gourd,** and **Indian gooseberry**.
- Zinc-rich foods: **Cashew nuts, sesame seeds, chickpeas,** and **oats**.
- Monounsaturated fats rich foods: **Olive oil** and **dry fruits**.
- Foods that increase fat-burning hormone adiponectin in the body: **Olive oil, chickpeas,** and **green peas**.
- Foods that reduce oxidative stress in the body and control diabetic complications: **Indian gooseberry**.

INSTANT AMLA PICKLE

Makes: 350 g | Prep time: 15 mins | Cooking time: 15 mins | Condiment

Ingredients

Indian gooseberry: 250 g	Fresh turmeric: 100 g
Kala namak mix: 1 tbsp	Asafoetida: ½ tsp
Mustard oil: 2 tbsp	

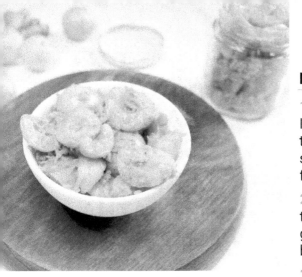

Method

1. Stream whole Indian gooseberries. Let them cool. Remove seeds. Peel and grate fresh turmeric.

2. Take grated turmeric and Indian gooseberry pieces in a bowl.

3. Add asafoetida, kala namak mix and mustard oil. Mix well.

4. Cover the bowl with a muslin cloth. Keep it in the sunlight for a day. Take it inside in the evening.

5. Fill Instant Amla Pickle in an airtight glass container. Store it under refrigeration for up to 2 weeks.

AMLA CHUTNEY

Makes: 120 g | Prep time: 10 mins
Condiment

Ingredients

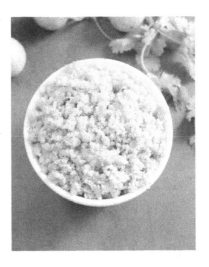

Indian gooseberry: 100 g	Green chili: 1
Coriander leaves: 25 g	Garlic: 7-8 cloves
Kala namak mix: 1 tbsp	

Method

1. Remove seeds from Indian gooseberry. Put all ingredients in a grinder jar.

2. Add coriander leaves Grind the chutney coarsely without adding water.

3. Enjoy the tangy Amla Chutney as it is or with rice and dal.

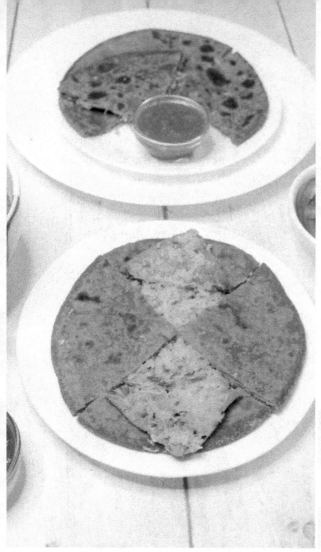

WHITE RADISH STUFFED PALAK PARATHA

Serves: 4 | Prep time: 20 mins | Cooking time: 20 mins | Breakfast

Ingredients

For Stuffing

Chopped green garlic: 50 g	White radish: 500 g
Chopped coriander leaves: 50 g	Cumin seeds: 1 tsp
Chopped ginger: 1 tsp	Salt: To taste
Asafoetida: ½ tsp	

For Tadka

Whole wheat flour: 400 g	Spinach: 200 g
Salt: To taste	Lemon juice: 1 tbsp
Olive oil: 1 tbsp + for making paratha	

Method

For Stuffing

1. Wash white radish thoroughly. Peel and grate them. Sprinkle salt over grated radish. Cover and keep aside for 15 minutes.

2. Squeeze radish to remove water. Take out as much water as you can. Keep the water for kneading.

3. Dry roast cumin seeds and crush them in a mortar with the help of a pestle.

4. Add cumin seeds, ginger, asafetida, green garlic, and coriander leaves to grated radish. Mix well and keep aside.

For Paratha

1. Blanch the spinach with lemon juice and salt for 1 to 2 minutes using minimal water. Make a fine paste by blending the spinach with the stock.

2. Add spinach paste and oil to whole wheat flour. Knead to a regular dough using radish water (if required). Cover and leave for 15 minutes.

3. Take a medium-sized ball from the dough. Make a smooth crack-free ball using your palms. Flatten the dough in your palm with your fingers. Keep center part a little thicker and sides thinner.

4. Put a spoonful of radish stuffing in the center, seal the edges, and make a smooth round ball. Flatten it gently with fingers. Dip it in dry whole wheat flour, dust off the excess flour.

5. Use a rolling pin to roll the dough into a circle.

6. Heat the pan/griddle/skillet (Tawa) on medium-high flame. Place the paratha on the skillet. Cook for about a minute or cook until the paratha begins puffing up from the base at some places.

7. Flip the paratha and spread 3-4 drops of olive oil. Cook for 2 minutes until it turns light brown.

8. Flip the paratha again and pour 3-4 drops of olive oil on top, and spread it evenly over the surface. Gently press the paratha with the flat spatula to help the paratha cook evenly.

9. When brown spots appear on both sides of the paratha, take out the paratha on a serving plate. Your paratha is ready. Similarly, make all the parathas.

10. Enjoy White radish stuffed Spinach Paratha with red and green chutney.

MULTIGRAIN METHI PURI

Makes: 165 g | Prep time: 30 mins | Cooking time: 15 mins | Snack

Ingredients

Oat flour: 75 g	Whole wheat flour: 75 g
Semolina: 15 g	Turmeric powder: 1 tsp
Asafoetida: A pinch	Salt: To taste
Extra virgin olive oil: 1 tbsp	Garam masala: 1 tbsp

To Grind Together

Peanuts: 70 g	Onion: 2 medium
Ginger: 1 inch	Sprouted fenugreek seeds: 2 tbsp
Cloves: 5	Green chilies: 2
Fennel: 1 tbsp	White sesame seeds: 2 tbsp
Curd: 1 tbsp, if required	Lemon juice: 1½ tbsp

Method

1. Dry roast peanuts. Remove from heat. Rub the peanuts between your palms to remove the skin.

2. Grind together peanuts, onion, ginger, cloves, chilies, fennel, sesame, sprouted fenugreek seeds, and lemon juice.

3. Take all three flours in a bowl. Add asafoetida, oil, salt, turmeric powder, garam masala, and mix well.

4. Add the prepared white paste to the flour mix and knead to make a slightly stiff dough. Add curd (if required).

5. Pinch a large ball from dough. Roll to a big round puri of (around 3 mm thick). Meanwhile, pre-heat the oven to 180 °C.

6. Take a fork and prick the surface of the puri so that it does not puff up while baking. Cut the puris into the desired shape with a cookie cutter. Repeat the process for rest of the dough.

7. Place the puris in a greased baking tray. Brush the puri top with oil. Bake puris in a pre-heated oven at 180 °C for 10 minutes. Flip the puris and bake for 5 minutes.

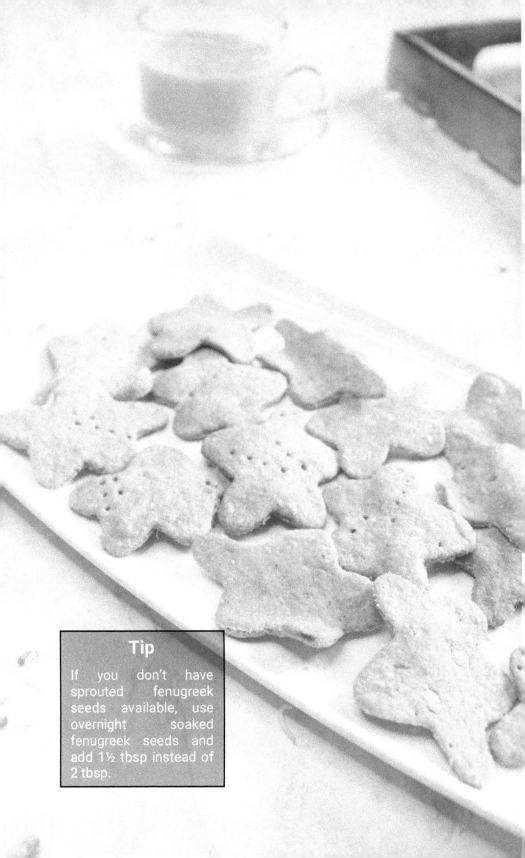

Tip

If you don't have sprouted fenugreek seeds available, use overnight soaked fenugreek seeds and add 1½ tbsp instead of 2 tbsp.

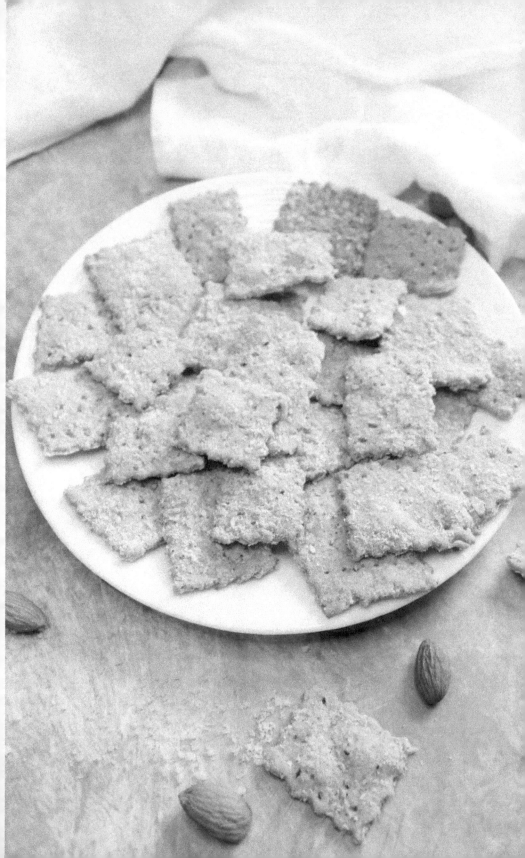

ALMOND CRACKERS

Makes: 150 g | Prep time: 15 mins | Cooking time: 15 mins | Snack

Ingredients

Whole wheat flour: 100 g

Oat flour: 50 g

Almond: 45 g

Desiccated coconut: 25 g

Salt: 1 tsp/to taste

Water: 75-100 ml

For Topping

White sesame seeds: 1 tbsp

Almond powder: 1 tbsp

Desiccated coconut: 1 tbsp

Method

1. Dry roast almonds till they slightly change color. Cool and grind to make a fine powder. Save 1 tbsp of almond powder for the topping and use the rest for dough.

2. Take whole wheat flour, oat flour, desiccated coconut, almond powder, and salt in a bowl. Gradually add water and knead to a stiff dough. The dough should not be soft. Leave covered for 10 minutes.

3. Pinch large size ball from the dough. Sprinkle flour to your work surface and roll the dough using a rolling pin to thickness to 3 mm to 4 mm. Cut out the sides with a cutter to make large rectangular dough sheet. Take a fork and prick it into the rolled dough to prevent the crackers to puff up while baking.

4. Sprinkle sesame seeds, almond powder, and desiccated coconut over dough sheet. Tap with your so that the nuts and seeds stick to the dough firmly.

5. With a zig-zag cutter or regular knife, cut the dough sheet to make 1 inch or 2 inches crackers.

6. Placed the crackers on the baking tray and bake in a pre-heated oven at 180 °C for 10 minutes. Flip the crackers and bake for 5 minutes or until the edges are browned.

7. Take out the crackers from the oven and allow them to cool completely before filling them in a container.Store in an airtight container and consume within 5 days.

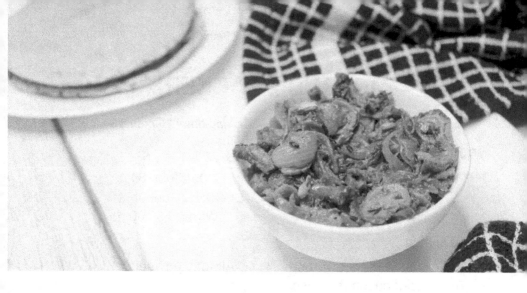

PYAZ WALE KARELE

Serves: 4 | Prep time: 15 mins | Cooking time: 30 mins | Side dish

Ingredients

Bitter gourd: 250 g	Onion: 200 g
Dry mango powder: ½ tsp	Cumin seeds: ½ tsp
Panch phoran masala: 1 tsp	Asafoetida: ¼ tsp
Salt: To taste	Oil: 2 tbsp

Method

1. Wash and soak bitter gourds in salted hot water for 15 minutes to reduce their bitterness. Dry them thoroughly with a kitchen towel. Remove both ends and peel them but do not throw the peel (see tip).Slice them. Cut onion lengthwise.

2. Add asafoetida and cumin seeds in hot oil. Cook for a minute. Add bitter gourds and cook on low flame for 15 minutes till they become crispy. Add onions and cook for 10 minutes.

3. Add panch phoran masala, dry mango powder and salt. Cook for 5 minutes. Serve hot.

Tip: Take the peel. of bitter gourd in a muslin cloth. Squeeze to collect bitter gourd juice. Discard the solid part and drink the juice while it is fresh. The juice will thicken if you keep it for later.

MUNG LITTI CHOKHA

Serves: 4 | Prep time: 30 mins | Cooking time: 50 mins | Main course (Weekend special)

Ingredients

For Dough

Whole wheat flour: 500 g

Water: To knead

Salt: To taste

Oil: 1 tbsp

For Mung Stuffing

Mung beans: 300 g

Turmeric powder: ½ tsp

Black pepper powder: ¼ tsp

Salt: To taste

Oil: 1 tsp

Cumin seeds: 1 tsp

Dried red chilies: 2

Asafoetida: ½ tsp

Water: 200 ml

For Chokha

Sweet potato: 150 g

Garlic: 8

Chopped coriander: 2 tbsp

Tomato: 3 medium

Chopped green chilies: 1

Salt: To taste

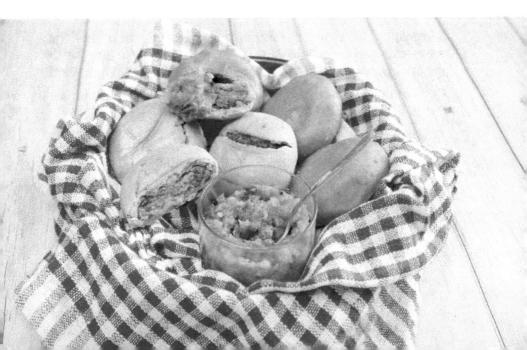

Method

For Dough

1. Mix all ingredients except water. Gradually add water and knead to a soft dough. Cover and leave for 30 minutes.

For Mung Stuffing

1. Soak mung beans in enough water overnight. Wash the overnight soaked mung beans with fresh water.
2. Heat oil in a pressure cooker. Add asafoetida, cumin seeds, and dried red chilies. Cook till cumin seeds change color.
3. Add mung beans. Cook for 5 minutes. Add turmeric powder, black pepper powder, and salt. Cook for 5 minutes.
4. Add water and pressure cook for 4 whistles on low flame. Mung beans should be completely cooked.
5. Mash the mung beans well with a masher or a pestle.
6. Return the cooker to heat and cook on low flame until all water evaporates and the stuffing dries up. Keep stirring it continuously to prevent the stuffing from sticking to the bottom of the cooker.

For Mung Litti

1. Take a medium-sized ball from the dough. Flatten the dough on your palm with your fingers. Keep center part a little thick and sides thin.
2. Fill a spoonful of mung stuffing in the center and seal the sides and make a ball. Gently press and flatten the litti. Brush the littis with oil and steam them in a steamer for 15 minutes.
3. Or bake the littis in a pre-heated oven at 200 °C for 10 minutes. Flip the littis and bake for 10-15 minutes.

For Chokha

1. Steam the sweet potatoes. Place the tomatoes and steamed sweet potatoes on a metal rack on a stove-top over direct flame. Roast from all sides till tomatoes are tender
2. Remove tomato and sweet potato skin and mash them.
3. Add crushed garlic, salt, chopped green chilies, and coriander leaves. Mix well and serve with Mung Littti.

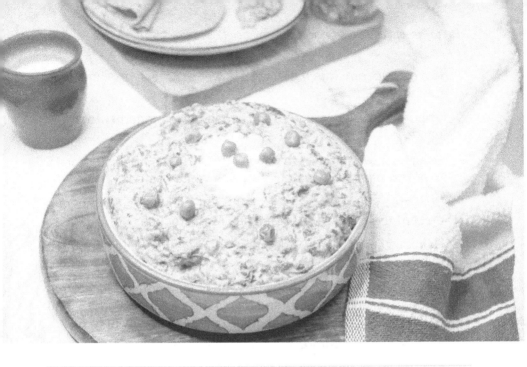

METHI MATAR IN WHITE GRAVY

Serves: 4 | Prep time: 30 mins | Cooking time: 50 mins | Main course (Weekend special)

Ingredients

Fresh fenugreek leaves: 200 g	Green peas: 100 g
Onion: 4 medium	Ginger: 1 inch
Garlic: 10	Green chilies: 2-3
Fresh curd: 200 g	Cashew nuts: 50 g
Melon seeds: 2 tbsp	Cumin seeds: ½ tsp
Bay leaf: 1	Asafoetida: ¼ tsp
Garam masala: 1 tsp	Coriander powder: ½ tsp
Salt: To taste	Water: 200 ml + as required
Ghee: 1½ tbsp	

Method

1. Chop fenugreek leaves. Sprinkle salt, cover, and leave for 15 minutes. Fenugreek leaves will release water. Squeeze out all the water. This step will reduce the bitterness of fenugreek

leaves. Do not throw fenugreek water. Use it for kneading dough.

2. Grind onion, ginger, garlic, and green chilies together to a fine paste.

3. Soak cashew nuts and melon seeds in 100 ml hot water for 15 minutes. Blend with water into a fine white paste.

4. Boil green peas in salted water for 5 minutes. Strain and discard the water. Keep green peas for later use.

5. Heat 1 tsp of ghee. Add fenugreek leaves. Cook for 8-10 minutes.

6. Meanwhile, heat 1 tbsp of ghee in another pan. Add asafoetida, cumin seeds, and bay leaf. Cook for a minute. Add onion paste. Cover and cook for 15 minutes on low flame.

7. Add cashew-melon paste. Cover and cook for 15 minutes on low flame. Stir occasionally.

8. Beat the curd with a spatula until smooth. Keep the flame low. Add curd. Cook for 5 minutes.

9. Add garam masala, coriander powder, and salt. Mix well. Cover and cook on low flame for 10 minutes or till the gravy leave oil. You will see the oil on top of the gravy.

10. Add 150 ml water (add more water if required). Bring it to a boil. Turn the flame to low and add fenugreek leave and green peas. Mix well. Simmer for 5 minutes on low flame. Serve hot with chapati and rice.

Tips

1. Use only fresh curd; otherwise, the gravy will turn sour. Another way to reduce the sourness of curd is to cook it well. The longer you cook the curd, the less sour it will be.

2. Always cook curd on low flame. Cooking on high flame may curdle the curd.

3. Adjust the amount of water according to taste. Gravy thickens with time. If your gravy has become thick, then add 50 ml-100 ml hot water and bring it to a boil.

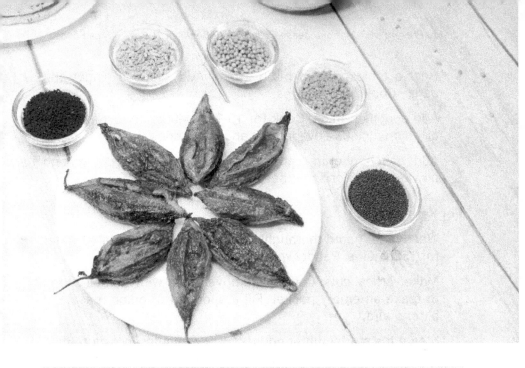

KARELA KALONJI

Serves: 4 | Prep time: 30 mins | Cooking time: 30 mins | Main course (Weekend special)

Ingredients

Bitter gourd: 10 small

Mustard oil: 1½ tbsp

Salt: To taste

For Stuffing

Garlic: 1 whole bulb (22-25 cloves)

Onion: 5 medium

Panch phoran masala: 1 tbsp

Ginger: 1 inch

Dry mango powder: ¼ tsp

Red chili powder: ¼ tsp

Mustard oil: 1 tbsp

Salt: To taste

Method

For Stuffing

1. Finely chop the onion, ginger and garlic.

2. Heat a tablespoon of oil in a pan. Add chopped ginger and garlic. Cook for 2 minutes.

3. Add chopped onion. Cook for 10-15 minutes on low flame till all onion moisture evaporates and onion dries up.

4. Add panch phoran, salt, red chili powder, and dry mango powder. Cook for 5 minutes. Keep aside.

For Karela Kalonji

1. Wash bitter gourd thoroughly and soak in hot and salted water for 15 minutes. Pat dry with a kitchen towel. Peel them.

2. Make vertical cuts. Carefully remove seeds with a small spoon to make an empty pocket. Fill a spoonful of onion masala in bitter gourd.

3. Steam the stuffed bitter gourds for 5-7 minutes, not more than that. This step is very important as it reduces 80% of the oil absorption of bitter gourds.

4. Heat a tablespoon of oil in a pan. Add 6-7 stuffed bitter gourds. Cover and cook for 15 minutes. Turn the bitter gourd every 3-4 minutes for even cooking. Cook till they are brown.

5. Once cooked, take out the bitter gourds from the pan. Add a teaspoon of oil and cook the rest of the stuffed bitter gourds.

6. Enjoy Karela Kaloji with chapati along with rice and dal in the afternoon on holiday, and you will not feel hungry till evening.

Tip

Cook the onion masala on low flame only. This may take longer, but it is an important step. Cooking the masala on low flame for a long time increases its sweetness and also enhances the taste.

NON-FRIED OATS BHATURE

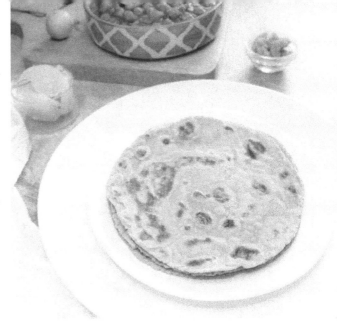

Serves: 4
Prep time: 10 mins
Cooking time: 20 mins
Main course

Ingredients

Oat flour: 300 g	Whole wheat flour: 200 g
Salt: To taste	Baking powder: ½ tsp
Curd: 250 g/as required	Olive oil: 1 tbsp + as required

Method

1. Take oat flour and whole wheat flour in a large bowl. Add salt, baking powder, and oil. Mix well.

2. Gradually add curd and knead for 5-6 minutes. The dough should be a little stiff for making crispy bhature. Add more curd if required.Cover the dough with a wet muslin cloth. Leave it for 3 hours.

3. Grease your palm well with oil. Take a medium size ball of dough and make a ball shape between your palms. Smooth out the ball, make sure it is crack-free. Roll it into oval shape or round disc.

4. Heat a Tawa/skillet. Grease it with oil and put bhatura on it. First, cook from one side. Spread ½ tsp of oil on top surface of bhatura. Turn and cook the other side. When brown spots appear on both sides, it's done. Eat Non-Fried Oats Bhature with chole masala.

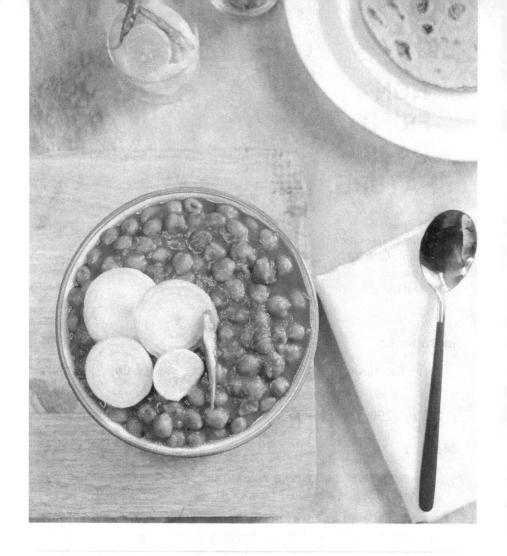

CHOLE MASALA

Serves: 4 | Prep time: 15 mins | Cooking time: 50 mins | Main course (Weekend Special)

Ingredients

To Cook Chickpeas

Uncooked dried Chickpeas: 400 g

Onion: 1 medium

Water: 1200 ml

Tea bags: 4

Salt: To taste

For Gravy

Garlic: 1 bulb/25-28 cloves	Ginger: 2 inches
Onion: 6 medium	Asafoetida: 1 tsp
Cumin seeds: 1 tsp	Bay leaves: 2
Red chili powder: ½ tsp	Turmeric powder: ½ tsp
Chole masala: 2 tbsp	Garam masala: 1 tsp
Water: 300 ml	Dry mango powder: 1 tsp
Mustard oil: 2 tbsp	Salt: To taste

Method

1. Soak the chickpeas in water overnight or for at least 8 hours. Next day, drain the water and rinse chickpeas thoroughly.

2. Take the soaked chickpeas, tea bags, salt, sliced onion (1 medium), and 1200 ml water in a pressure cooker. Pressure cook on medium flame for 5-6 whistles. It will take around 15 minutes. Check if chickpeas are hard, then pressure cook them for two whistles.

3. Squeeze and discard the tea bags. Strain the chickpeas and keep the stock for later use. Grind onion, garlic, and ginger to make a smooth paste.

4. Add mustard oil to the hot pan. Add asafoetida, cumin seeds, and bay leaves, and sauté for 2 minutes.

5. Add the onion paste to the oil. Mix well and cover and cook on medium-low flame for 15 minutes. Cook till it leaves oil.

6. Add chole masala, garam masala, turmeric powder, dry mango powder, red chili powder, and salt. Cook for 5 minutes.

7. Add chickpeas and mix well. Masala mixture should coat the chickpeas entirely. Cook for 5-7 minutes.

8. Add the chickpeas stock plus 300 ml of water. Don't add too much water as it will dilute the taste.Bring it to a boil. Turn the flame to low. Cook for 10 minutes until chickpeas absorb the flavor of masala. The gravy should be thick.

9. Your Chole Masala is ready to eat. Eat it with non-fried oats bhature or brown rice.

ANJEER KAJU KATLI

Zinc deficiency may lead to the development of diabetes. Zinc plays an important role in preventing and managing diabetes. It is because zinc plays a crucial part in the production and secretion of insulin. Since zinc strengthens the immune system, it protects beta cells from destruction. Studies suggest that zinc-rich foods help lower blood sugar levels in type 1 as well as type 2 diabetes. Cashew nuts are a great source of zinc. This sweet is all about cashew nuts and requires less sweetness as compared to other sweets. The milder the sweetness, the richer cashew nuts will taste.

Makes: 200 g | Prep time: 20 mins | Cooking time: 15 mins | Dessert

Ingredients

Cashew nuts: 200 g	Dried figs: 22
Water: 180 ml	Ghee: For greasing
Edible silver leaves/vark: 3 or 4	

Method

1. Wash and soak figs in 180 ml water for 2 hours.

2. Take figs along with water in a pressure cooker. Pressure cook for 3-4 whistles. Turn off the flame. Let it cool down. Blend it in a blender to make a fine paste. Make sure the paste is smooth.

3. Take the paste in a muslin cloth. Squeeze to collect the smooth fig paste. Discard the solid part. Alternatively, you can pass it through a sieve and discard the solid part.

4. Finely grind cashew nuts. Pass through a sieve and grind the coarse nuts again to make a fine powder.

5. Take the fig paste in a pan. Bring it to a boil. Cook till it reduces to one-fourth of the volume and the water has almost evaporated.

6. When the fig paste starts separating from the pan, add cashew powder. Mix well and keep stirring continuously so that it does not stick to the bottom of the pan. Keep the flame medium.

228

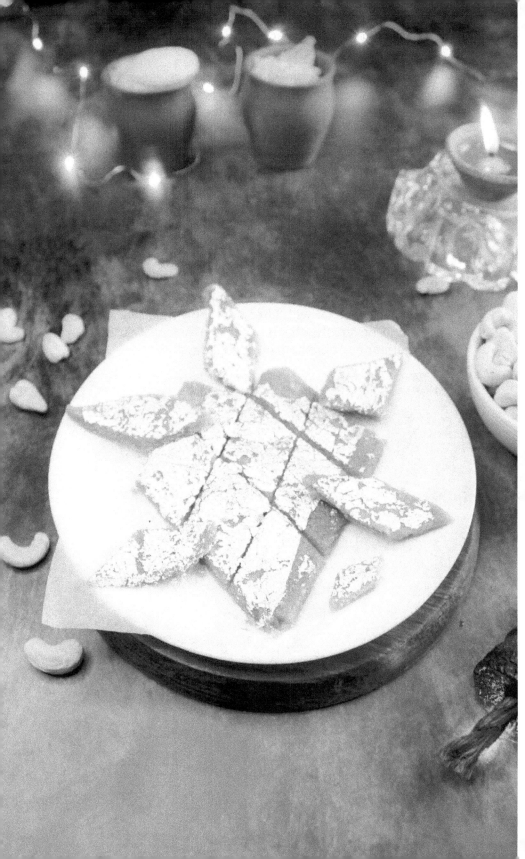

7. Cook till mixture comes together and releases oil. You will notice oil around the mixture, and it will start separating from the pan. It takes around 3-5 minutes to reach this stage. Turn off the flame.

8. Take out the mixture on a well-greased bowl or plate. Let it cool down for 5 minutes. It will dry out and look like dough.

9. Knead the anjeer kaju katli dough for 3 minutes.

10. Place the dough on butter paper, place another butter paper over it, and flatten the dough into a thickness of 3 to 5 mm with a rolling pin.

11. Remove the butter paper from the top. Apply silver vark while the kaju katli is still hot. If the anjeer kaju katli has become cold, then grease it with ghee and apply the silver vark. Cut in diamond or square shape. Keep the Anjeer Kaju Katli in the refrigerator and consume it within 3 days.

Tips

1. Do not grind cashews at high speed or for a long time, or else it will start releasing oil which is not good for this recipe.

2. Do not add extra water than what is mentioned in the recipe. The fig paste may seem thick and less initially, but it is enough to make the perfect anjeer kaju katli. If you add more water, katli will become sticky and will not dry out later and look like halwa.

3. Applying silver vark is optional. Traditionally Kaju Katli has silver vark, but it is completely optional. Make sure to check the product label. It should clearly specify that it's 100% vegetarian or confirm with the seller if the silver vark is 100% vegetarian. When in doubt, omit silver vark completely.

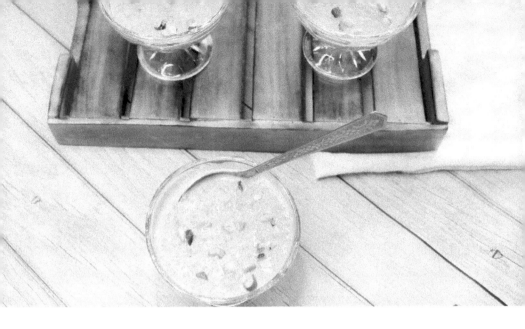

LAUKI KI KHEER

Serves: 4 | Prep time: 20 mins | Cooking time: 40 mins | Dessert

Ingredients

Bottle gourd: 200 g	Milk: 1 L
Dates: 11-13	Almonds: 8
Raisins: 10	Cashew nuts: 8
Ghee: 1 tbsp	Saffron: 5-6 strands

Method

1. Soak saffron in 2 tbsp of hot milk. Keep aside. Remove seeds from dates and blend them with 50 ml of milk. Keep aside.

2. Peel and grate bottle gourd (remove seeds). Heat ghee in a pan. Add the grated bottle gourd and cook for 5-8 minutes. Bottle gourd should be cooked well, or it might curdle the milk.

3. Bring milk to a boil. Cook on medium flame till the milk thickens slightly. Stir occasionally.Add bottle gourd. Cook for 20-25 minutes on medium flame.

4. Add date paste, saffron milk, chopped almond, cashew nuts, and raisins. The kheer will start thickening immediately. Simmer for 5 minutes on low flame. Turn off the flame.

5. Allow it to cool to room temperature, then refrigerate for 2-3 hours. Enjoy chilled Lauki ki Kheer.

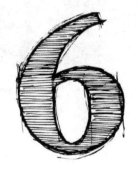

EAT

TO

PREVENT

AND

CONTROL

HYPERTENSION

Blood pressure is the measure of the force of blood against blood vessel walls. The blood pressure increases when the force of blood against the artery walls is too high, and this condition is known as hypertension or high blood pressure. To prevent and control hypertension, your diet should be rich in foods that have the following therapeutic effects:

- Foods that have diuretic effects.

- Foods that have potent vasodilating properties.

- Foods rich in magnesium as magnesium is a natural calcium channel blocker.

- Foods rich in potassium because potassium negates the sodium effect.

- Foods that keep nitric oxide levels high in your body.

Superfoods that prevent and control hypertension are:

Vasodilator: **Beetroot** and **garlic**.

Diuretics: **Cucumber** and **lemon**.

Magnesium-rich foods: **Spinach, kidney beans, pumpkin seeds, pistachios,** and **sweet potato**.

Potassium-rich foods: **Cucumber, sweet potato, kidney beans, banana, spinach,** and **curd**.

Foods that increase nitric oxide production in the body: **Beetroot, honey,** and **pumpkin seeds**.

This chapter helps you include superfoods in your diet that help prevent and manage hypertension effectively.

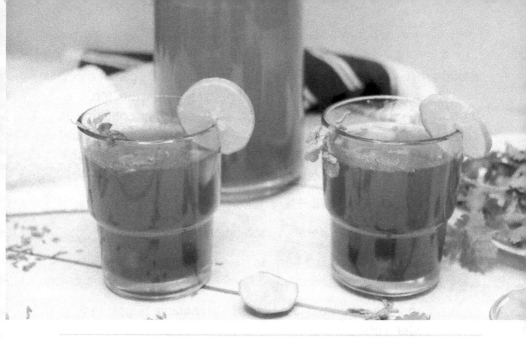

CUCUMBER JALJEERA

Serves: 4 | Prep time: 15 mins | Cooking time: 5 mins | Beverage

Ingredients

Lemon juice: 2 tbsp	Mint leaves: 50 g
Coriander leaves: 30 g	Ginger: 1½ inches
Green chili: 1	Cumin seeds: 1 tsp
Dried mango powder: ½ tsp	Asafoetida: ½ tsp
Black salt: To taste	Black pepper: 10
Cloves: 4	Cucumber pieces: 4 tbsp
Water: 1 L	

Method

1. Dry roast cumin seeds, cloves, and black pepper till cumin seeds turn reddish-brown. Cool and grind them.

2. Finely chop the cucumber. Keep aside for later.

3. Take all the ingredients in the blender jar except the cucumber. Add about 50 ml - 100 ml of water and grind to a-fine paste.

4. Take the green paste in a jar and add more water to make 1 L. Add cucumber pieces. Refrigerate it for 2 hours. Serve chilled.

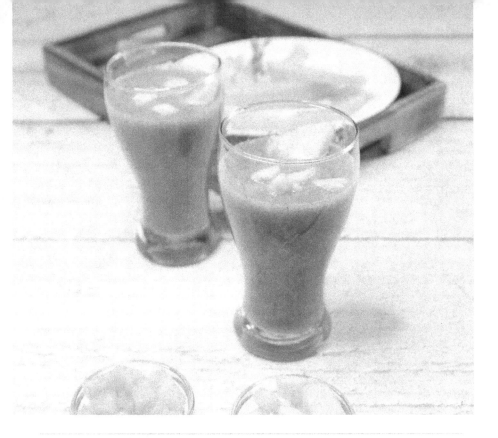

SUMMER FRUIT PUNCH

Serves: 4 | Prep time: 15 mins | Beverage

Ingredients

Musk melon: 500 g	Cucumber: 250 g
Orange: 200 g	Mint leaves: 50 g
Honey: 1 tbsp/To taste	Lemon juice: 1 tbsp
Dry mango powder: 1 tsp	Ice cubes: 8-10 (optional)

Method

1. Chill musk melon, cucumber, orange, and mint leaves in the refrigerator for 3-4 hours.

2. Keep 4-5 mint leaves to garnish. Blend musk melon, cucumber, orange and mint leaves, lemon juice, and honey in a blender.

3. Pour the fruit punch into glasses. Sprinkle dry mango powder over it. If you want, put 2-3 ice cubes in each glass. Enjoy the chilled and refreshing Summer Fruit Punch.

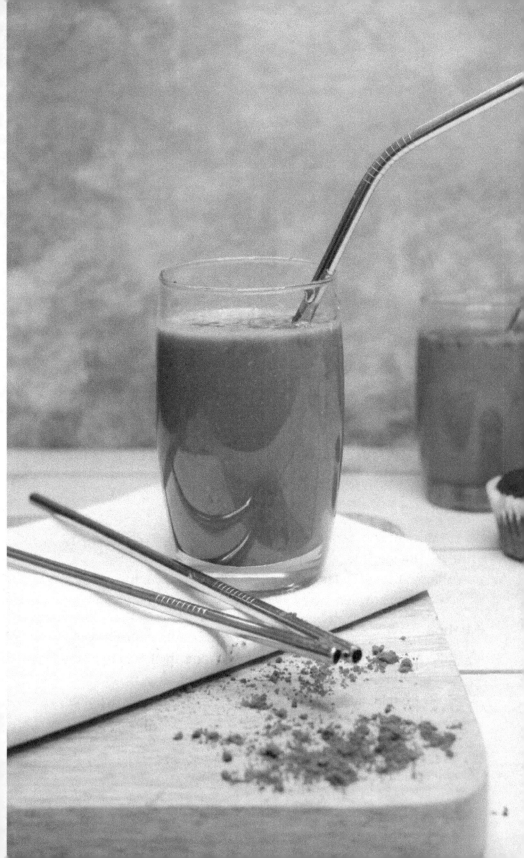

BANANA CHOCO MILK SHAKE

Serves: 4 | Prep time: 15 mins | Beverage

Ingredients

Banana: 4

Cocoa powder: 1 tbsp

Pistachios: 2 tbsp

Chilled cow milk: 800 ml

Honey: 1 tbsp (optional)

Pumpkin seeds: 1 tbsp

Method

1. Dry roast pistachios and pumpkin seeds till they start releasing an aromatic smell and turn slightly brown. Remove from flame and let the nuts cool down. Chop them roughly using a knife or crush them using the mortar pestle or grinder.

2. Chop banana roughly. Blend banana, cocoa powder, and chilled milk into a smooth milkshake. Pour into glasses and add honey if needed.

3. Add pistachios and pumpkin seeds. Mix well and serve.

CRISPI GARLICI SWEET POTATO

Serves: 4 | Prep time: 15 mins | Cooking time: 20 mins | Snack

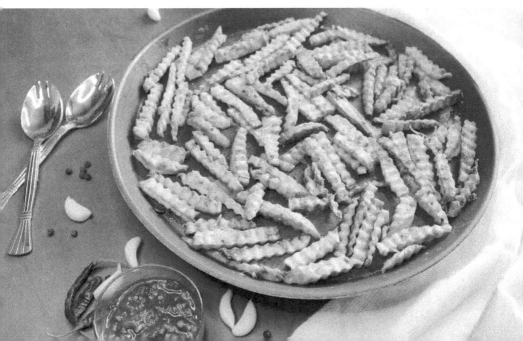

Ingredients

Sweet potato: 600 g	Rock salt: To taste
Kashmiri red chili powder: 1 tbsp	Black pepper powder: 1 tsp
Garlic: 15-18 cloves	Oil: 2½ tbsp
Corn flour: 1 tbsp	Dry mango powder: ½ tsp

Method

1. Wash and peel sweet potatoes (or leave the skin on). Cut them with a zig-zag knife or simple knife to medium thickness.

2. Steam sweet potatoes in a steamer for 5 minutes, not more than that.

3. Crush garlic finely using mortar pestle. Add Kashmiri red chili powder, salt, black pepper powder, and oil. Mix well.

4. Take out sweet potatoes in a colander. Add corn flour and toss to coat sweet potatoes evenly.

5. Add the garlic seasoning. Toss until sweet potatoes are evenly coated with the seasoning and don't look dry.

6. Divide sweet potatoes into 2 batches. Place one batch on a greased baking dish.

7. If you have the grill function in your oven, grill sweet potatoes for 12 minutes. Flip the sides and grill for 3-5 minutes.

8. Alternatively, bake the sweet potatoes in a pre-heated oven at 200 °C for 15 minutes. Flip the sides for even cooking and bake for 5-10 minutes or until sweet potatoes are crisp and browned from corners.

9. Take them out from the oven. Sprinkle dry mango powder and enjoy Crispi Garlici Sweet Potato with bell pepper chutney.

Tip

Steaming sweet potatoes shortens the baking time and prevents the sweet potatoes from releasing sugar. Cooking in this way makes sweet potatoes even more healthy.

MULTIGRAIN BEETROOT PARATHA

Serves: 4 | Prep time: 15 mins | Cooking time: 20 mins | Breakfast

Ingredients

Grated beetroot: 150 g	Grated bottle gourd: 150 g
Whole wheat flour: 150 g	Oat flour: 150 g
Gram flour/chickpea flour: 75 g	Salt: To taste
Amaranth flour: 25 g	Coriander powder: 1 tsp
Ginger garlic paste: 1 tbsp	Red chili powder: 1 tsp
Jaggery: 1 tbsp	Turmeric powder: ½ tsp
Garam masala: 1½ tsp	Sesame seeds: 1½ tbsp
Asafoetida: a pinch	Olive oil: 1 tbsp+ as needed
Crushed fenugreek seeds: 1 tsp	Curd: 2 tbsp (to knead)

Method

1. Take all ingredients along with one tbsp of olive oil in a bowl. Gradually add curd and knead to a stiff dough.

2. Take a dough ball, dip it in the dry whole wheat flour, and dust off the excess flour. Use a rolling pin to roll the dough into a circle. Heat the griddle/skillet (Tawa) on medium-high flame.

3. Place the paratha on the skillet. Cook for about a minute or cook until the paratha begins puffing up from the base.

4. Flip the paratha and spread 3-4 drops of olive oil. Cook for 2 minutes until it turns light brown.

5. Flip the paratha again and top with

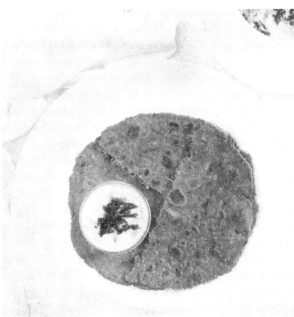

3-4 drops of olive oil, spread it evenly over the surface. Press the paratha gently with a flat spatula to cook paratha evenly.

6. Once you begin to see brown spots on both sides of the paratha, transfer the paratha to a serving plate. Your paratha is ready. Similarly, make all the parathas.

7. Enjoy Multigrain Beetroot Paratha with mixed veg raita.

MIXED VEG RAITA

Serves: 4 | Prep time: 15 mins | Side dish

Ingredients

Curd: 400 g	Grated beetroot: 2 tbsp
Finely chopped onion: 50 g	Finely chopped tomato: 50 g
Finely chopped cabbage: 50 g	Finely chopped cucumber: 50 g
Brown sugar: 1 tbsp	Kala namak mix: 1 tsp/to taste
Cumin seeds powder: 1 tbsp	Red chili powder: ½ tsp

Method

1. Blend the curd until smooth. Add all veggies except beetroot.

2. Add kala namak mix, brown sugar, red chili powder, and cumin seeds powder to the curd. Mix well.

3. Keep the raita in the fridge for half an hour. Garnish with grated beetroot. Enjoy it with multigrain beetroot paratha.

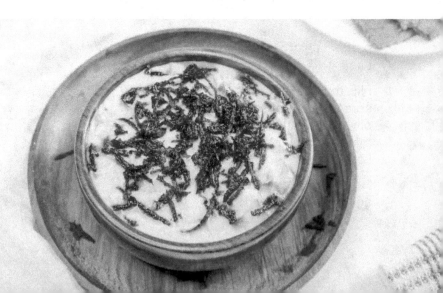

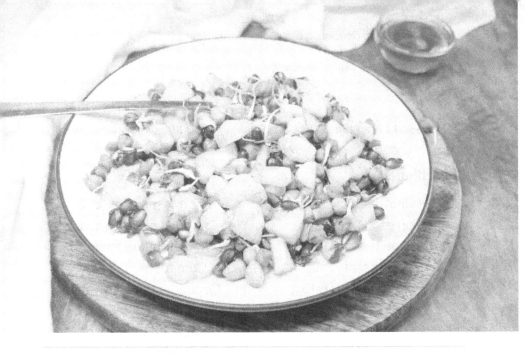

CUCUMBER SALAD

Serves: 4 | Prep time: 15 mins | Salad

Ingredients

Cucumber: 1 large	Banana: 1
Sprouted brown chickpeas: 3 tbsp	Pomegranate: 3 tbsp
Peanuts: 2 tbsp	Red chili powder: ½ tsp
Honey: 1 tsp	Lemon juice: 2 tbsp
Chopped mint leaves: 2 tbsp	Kala namak mix: To taste
Coriander leaves: 2 tbsp	

Method

1. Soak peanuts in water for 2 hours. Cut banana and cucumber into half-inch cubes.

2. Roughly chop mint leaves and coriander leaves.

3. Take all ingredients in a bowl and mix well. Cover and leave for 15 minutes until the lemon juice moistens the salad.

4. Enjoy the Cucumber Salad.

RAJMA

*Serves: 4 | Prep time: 15 mins | Cooking time: 30 mins | Main course
(Weekend special)*

Ingredients

Kidney beans: 300 g	Onion: 4 medium (1+3)
Tomato: 4 medium	Chopped ginger: 1 tbsp
Chopped garlic: 1 tbsp	Asafoetida: 1 tsp
Bay leaf: 1	Cumin seeds: ½ tsp
Garam masala: 1½ tbsp	Coriander powder: 1 tsp
Turmeric powder: ½ tsp	Red chili powder: 1 tsp
Salt: To taste	Mustard oil: 2 tbsp
Water: 900 ml	Coriander leaves: 20 g

Method

1. Soak kidney beans in enough water overnight.Cut onion lengthwise. Keep one onion for cooking kidney beans and the rest three for gravy.

2. Pressure cook kidney beans with one chopped onion, salt, and water for 3-4 whistle. Check whether the kidney beans are cooked; If not, pressure cook for 2 more whistles. Strain the cooked kidney beans and keep the stock for gravy.

3. Heat mustard oil in a pan. Once the oil is hot, add bay leaf, asafoetida, and cumin seeds.

4. When cumin seeds start changing color, add ginger and garlic and cook on medium flame for 2 minutes.

5. Add onions and cook for 6-8 minutes till onions turn translucent. Add chopped tomatoes and salt and mix well. Cover and cook on low flame for 10 minutes. Stir occasionally.

6. Add garam masala, coriander powder, red chili powder, turmeric powder. Cover and cook on low flame for 5 minutes.

7. Add kidney beans and cook for 5 minutes on medium flame. Add stock and bring to a boil. Pressure cook for 1-2 whistles.

8. Garnish with coriander leaves and enjoy Rajma with rice.

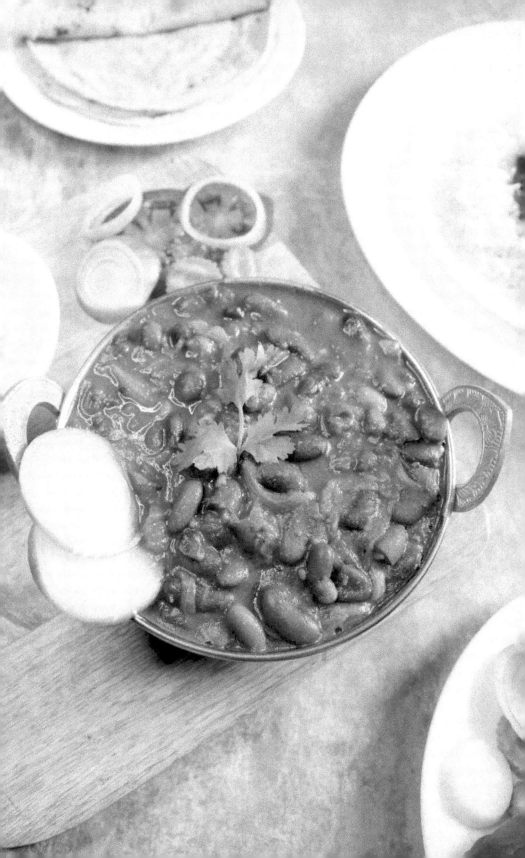

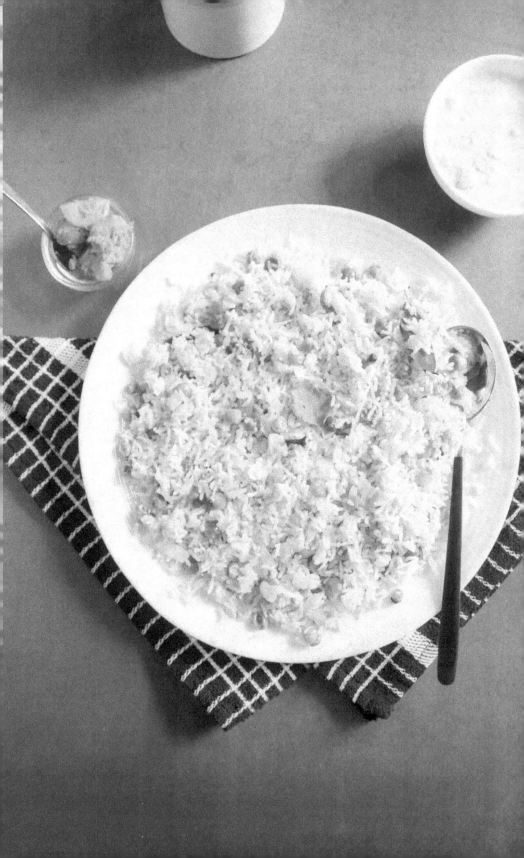

MIXED VEG PULAO

Serves: 4 | Prep time: 15 mins | Cooking time: 30 mins | Main course (Weekend special)

Ingredients

Basmati rice: 400 g	Peas: 150 g
Cabbage: 150 g	Carrot: 150 g
Cloves: 6	Black pepper: 10
Cinnamon: 1 inch	Green cardamom: 3
Cumin seeds: 1 tsp	Asafoetida: ½ tsp
Bay leaf: 1	Salt: To taste
Ghee: 2 tbsp	Water: 850 ml

Method

1. Wash rice in running water and soak rice for 15 minutes.

2. Chop cabbage and carrot.Crush clove, cardamom, cinnamon, and black pepper in a mortar with the help of a pestle.

3. Heat ghee in a pressure cooker. Add bay leaf, asafoetida, cumin seeds, crushed cloves, cinnamon, cardamom, and black pepper. Cook till cumin seeds start changing color.

4. Add peas and salt, cover and cook for 5 minutes till peas are tender. Add carrots and cook for 5 minutes without covering. Add cabbage and cook for 5 minutes without covering.

5. Strain the rice and add it to the vegetable mixture. Cook for 6-8 minutes. Stir occasionally to prevent rice from sticking at the bottom of the cooker. Do not stir vigorously; otherwise, the rice will break.

6. Add water and close the lid of the cooker. Cook on medium flame for 1 whistle. Turn off the flame. Leave for 5 minutes and open the lid. Do not keep the lid of the pressure cooker on for a long time; otherwise, the rice will be soggy.

7. Enjoy Mixed Veg Pulav as it is or with rajma or dal fry.

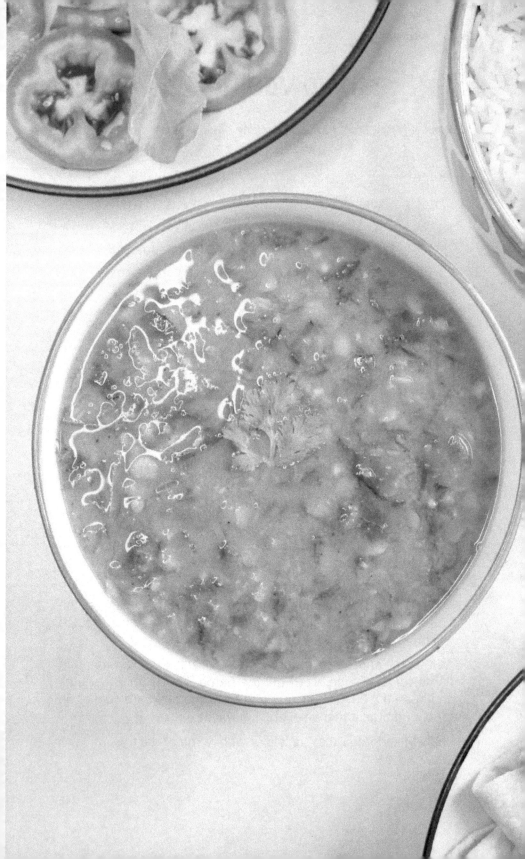

DAL FRY PALAK WALE

Serves: 4 | Prep time: 20 mins | Cooking time: 40 mins | Main course

Ingredients

Spinach: 200 g	Yellow split pigeon peas: 140 g
Split Bengal gram: 50 g	Salt: To taste
Water: 650 ml	Turmeric: ½ tsp

For Tadka

Ginger: 1 inch	Garlic: 6 cloves
Onion: 1 medium	Tomatoes: 1 medium
Garam masala: ½ tsp	Coriander powder: ½ tsp
Red chili powder ¼ tsp	Cumin seeds: ½ tsp
Asafoetida: ½ tsp	Oil: 1 tbsp
Water: 250 ml	

Method

1. Wash and chop spinach leaves. Wash split pigeon peas and split Bengal gram 2-3 times. Soak them in water for 15 mins.

2. Discard the water. Take dal in the pressure cooker, add fresh 650 ml water. Bring to a boil. Add salt, turmeric powder, and spinach leaves. Close the lid and pressure cook on a medium flame for 4 whistles.

3. Heat oil in a pan. Add asafoetida and cumin seeds. Cook till cumin seeds start changing color.Add chopped ginger and garlic and cook for 2 minutes. Add onion and cook for 5-7 minutes. Add tomato and salt. Cook for 5 minutes.

4. Add garam masala, coriander powder, and red chili powder. Cover and cook for 10 minutes. Mash the mix with a spatula.

5. Add dal to it and mix. Add 250 ml water, if required, add more water. Bring it to a boil. Cook on low flame for 5-10 minutes. Serve hot with rice.

Note: *Spinach absorbs less salt, due to which you will need less salt than usual, so add salt accordingly.*

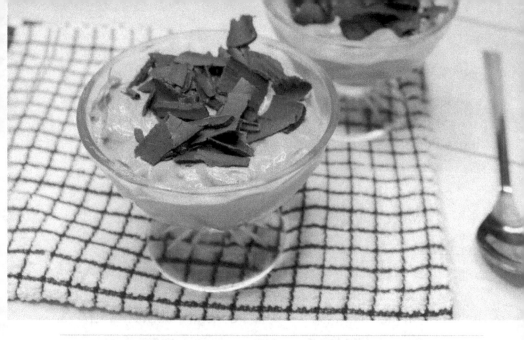

CHOCOLATE SHRIKHAND

Serves: 4 | Prep time: 12 hours | Dessert

Ingredients

Fresh thick curd: 2 L	Cocoa powder: 2 tbsp
Honey: To taste	Vanilla essence: ½ tsp
Dark chocolate pieces: 4 tbsp	Dark chocolate shaves: 2 tbsp

Method

1. Tie thick curd in a muslin cloth and hang it on a tap or any other place overnight or for 6-7 hours.

2. Take out the hung curd in a bowl. Blend it with a spoon or hand blender to make it smooth. Mix cocoa powder, honey, and vanilla essence in the hung curd.

3. Take shrikhand in a muslin cloth and pass the shrikhand through muslin cloth by squeezing the muslin cloth or pass the shrikhand through a sieve to make it smooth.

4. Add the chocolate pieces. Refrigerate it for 3-4 hours.

5. Take out Shrikhand in individual serving bowls. Decorate with chocolate shavings. Keep the bowl in the refrigerator for half an hour and enjoy Chocolate Shrikhand after lunch.

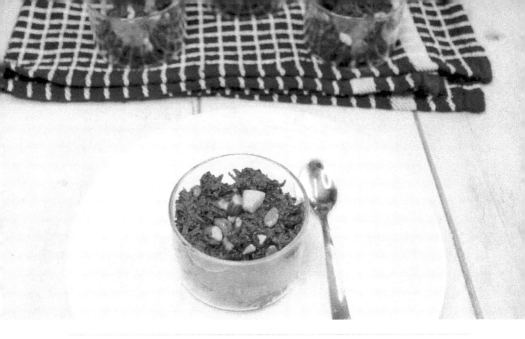

RED VELVET HALWA

Serves: 4 | Prep time: 10 mins | Cooking time: 30 mins | Dessert

Ingredients

Grated Beetroot: 300 g	Milk: 500 ml
Jaggery: 50 g	Desiccated coconut: 6 tbsp
Chopped mixed nuts: 2 tbsp	Ghee ½ tsp

Method

1. Heat ghee in a pan. Add chopped nuts and roast till they start releasing a pleasant aromatic smell. Make sure to stir continuously. Take out the nuts and keep them aside.

2. In the same pan, add milk and bring it to a boil. Keep boiling till the milk thickens slightly (about 5-7 minutes on high flame).

3. Add grated beetroot to the milk. Keep the flame medium-high and let it cook till all milk evaporates. Keep stirring it to prevent it from sticking to the pan. It will take about 15 to 20 minutes.

4. When the milk has reduced to about 90%, it will look like a slurry. Add jaggery and desiccated coconut at this stage.

5. Cook for 5 minutes till the beetroot absorbs all the milk and starts leaving the pan. Turn off the flame. Add all nuts and mix well. Serve hot or refrigerate for 3 hours before serving.

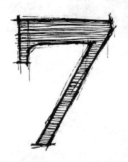

EAT TO PREVENT AND CONTROL ARTHRITIS

Arthritis is a joint disorder characterized by swelling with stiffness and joint pain. To prevent and control arthritis, your diet should be rich in foods that have the following activities:

- Foods that reduce inflammation.
- Foods that have potent antioxidant properties.

- Foods that modulate immune activity.
- Foods that balance the gut microbiome.

This chapter helps you include superfoods in your diet that have therapeutic effects and help prevent and manage arthritic conditions effectively.

Superfoods that prevent and control arthritis are:

- Foods that reduce inflammation in the body through their anti-inflammatory and antioxidant properties: **Turmeric, horse gram, walnuts, mushrooms,** and **licorice root**.
- Foods rich in omega-3 fatty acids: **Flax seeds, chia seeds,** and **soybean**.
- Foods rich in calcium: **Chia seeds, sesame,** and **soybean**.
- Foods rich in vitamin K: **Soybean, cabbage,** and **nuts**.
- Pre-biotics foods that increase the good bacteria and crowd out pro-inflammatory bacteria in the gut: **Oats, garlic, onion, soybean, flax seeds, almonds,** and **cocoa powder**.

Note: *1. Although soybeans are high in omega-3 fats, vitamin K, and calcium, all of which are important for bone health, they are also high in omega-6 fats that have pro-inflammatory effects when consumed in excess. Therefore, consume soybeans in moderation.*

2. Don't eat too much licorice, especially if your blood pressure is already high. Licorice in excess can increase blood pressure.

MULETHI HERBAL CHAI

Serves: 4 | Prep time: 5 mins | Cooking time: 15 mins | Beverage

Ingredients

Licorice root: 2 inches	Ashwagandha root: 2 inches
Cinnamon stick: 1 inch	Black Pepper: 8
Ginger: 1½ inches	Water: 800 ml

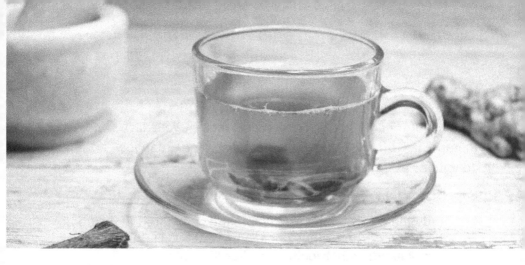

Method

1. Crush ginger, cinnamon, and black pepper using a pestle. Add these herbs, licorice root, and ashwagandha root in water.

2. Bring it to a boil. Simmer for 10 minutes on medium flame till water reduces to 600 ml.

3. Strain the tea. The licorice root is enough to make tea sweet (sweetener is not needed). Drink hot Mulethi Herbal Chai.

FENNEL CHIA SEEDS MILK SHAKE

Serves: 4 | Prep time: 30 mins | Cooking time: 10 mins | Beverage

Ingredients

Skimmed milk: 1 L	Fennel: 5 tbsp
Honey: If required	Almonds: 100 g
Water: 80 ml	Chia seeds: 2 tbsp

Method

1. Soak chia seeds in 80 ml water overnight or for at least 4 hrs.

2. Soak almonds in hot water for 30 minutes. Remove the skin and blend it with 50 ml milk to make a thick cream. Keep it in fridge for 2 hours.

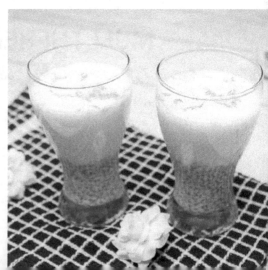

3. Wash the fennel seeds thoroughly. Dry on a kitchen towel for 20 minutes. Finely grind the fennel seeds.

4. Bring the milk to a boil. Turn the flame to low. Add fennel seeds powder and simmer for 5 minutes.

5. Turn off the flame and let it cool down. Strain the milk. Add honey, mix well and chill for 2 hours in the refrigerator.

6. Add almond cream into individual glasses. Add a spoonful of soaked chia seeds. Pour fennel milk and enjoy refreshing Fennel Chia Seeds Milk Shake.

GRILLED MUSHROOMS

Serves: 4 | Prep time: 10 mins | Cooking time: 15 mins | Snack

Ingredients

Button mushrooms: 600 g	Black pepper powder: 1 tsp
Red chili powder: ¼ tsp	Extra virgin olive oil: 2 ½ tbsp
Salt: To taste	

Method

1. Wash the mushrooms thoroughly and cut them into half an inch. Sprinkle salt, red chili powder, and black pepper powder.

2. Add oil and mix well. Spread the mushroom pieces on the baking tray. Make sure they do not overlap each other. If the quantity is more, grill/bake in 2 batches.

3. If you have grill function in your oven, grill mushrooms for 15 minutes or bake in a pre-heated oven at 180°C for 15 minutes.

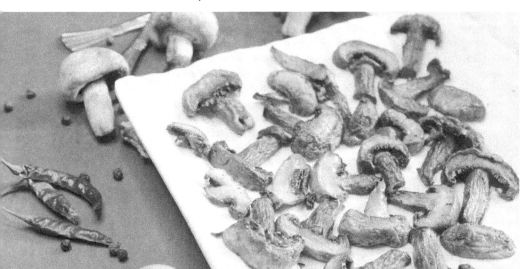

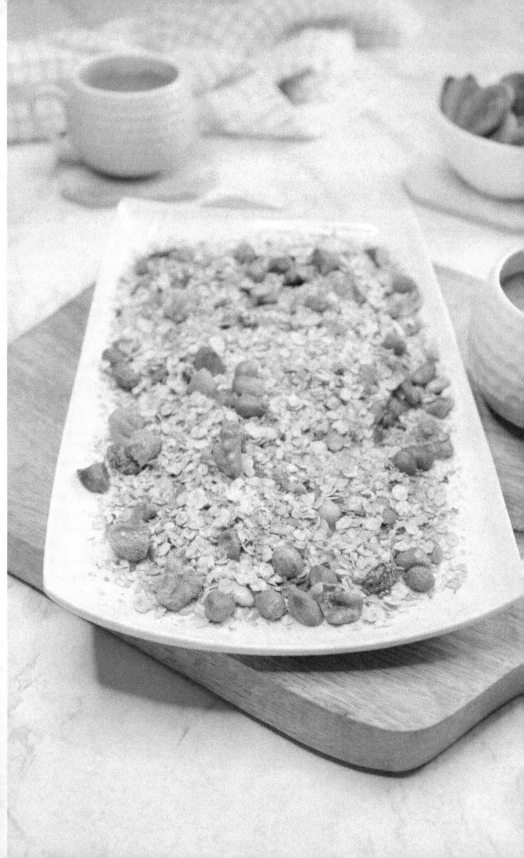

OATS WALNUT NAMKEEN

Makes: 300 g | Prep time: 10 mins | Cooking time: 20 mins | Snack

Ingredients

Rolled oats: 200 g	Walnuts: 40 g
Desiccated coconut: 25 g	Coriander seeds: 1 tbsp
Fennel: 1 tbsp	Curry leaves: 20-25
Sesame seeds: 2 tbsp	Peanuts: 35 g
Almonds: 12	Pistachios: 10
Pumpkin seeds: 2 tbsp	Raisins: 2 tbsp
Asafoetida: 1 tsp	Garam masala: ½ tsp
Turmeric powder: 1 tsp	Brown sugar: 1 ½ tbsp
Kashmiri red chili powder: 1 tbsp	Dry mango powder: 1 tsp
Salt: To taste	

Method

1. Chop walnuts, almonds, and pistachios. Dry roast fennel seeds and coriander seeds and desiccated coconut till they start releasing an aromatic smell. Grind them coarsely in a mixer grinder. Keep the masala for later use.

2. Dry roast oats till they start changing color. Keep it aside. Heat oil in a pan. Add asafoetida, sesame seeds and curry leaves in it and cook for a minute.

3. Add peanuts and roast for 5 minutes.Add almonds, pistachios, pumpkin seeds, walnuts, and raisins one by one. Roast till they turn slightly brown.

4. Add turmeric powder, chili powder, salt, garam masala, and dry mango powder. Cook for a minute.

5. Add roasted rolled oats. Mix well. Add prepared masala and brown sugar. Mix well.

6. Turn off the flame and leave the oats walnut namkeen in the pan till it cools down completely.

7. Enjoy Oats Walnut Namkeen with evening tea. Store the namkeen in an airtight container for up to 15 days.

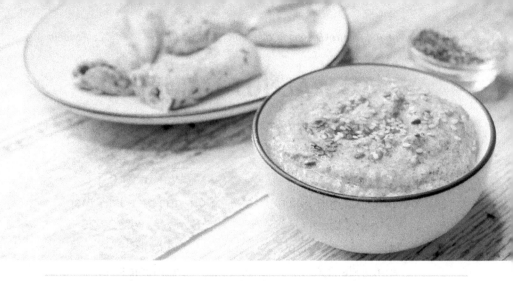

FLAX SEEDS SPREAD

Makes: 110 g | Prep time: 10 mins | Cooking time: 10 mins | Condiment

Ingredients

Flax seeds: 30 g	Sesame seeds: 30 g
Garlic: 15-18 cloves	Dry red chilies: 2
Cumin seeds: 3 tsp	Lemon juice: 3 tsp
Extra virgin olive oil: 1 tsp	Salt: To taste
Water: 60 ml	

Method

1. Dry roast flax seeds on low flame till flax seeds turn dark and slightly puffed up. Remove from heat.

2. Dry roast sesame seeds, cumin seeds, and red chilies till they slightly change color. Keep stirring it to prevent the burning.

3. Grind all the ingredients together except olive oil to make a superfine spread. Add extra virgin olive oil and mix.

4. Apply Flax Seeds Spread on toast or use as a dip or serve as chutney. Store it in the refrigerator and consume within 3 days.

Tip
Proper roasting of flax seeds is an important step to reduce the peculiar taste of flax seeds. The spread will taste bitter if the flax seeds are not roasted well, so roast them until they become slightly puffed.

MUSHROOM WALNUT SOUP

Serves: 4 | Prep time: 5 mins | Cooking time: 20 mins | Starter

Ingredients

Sliced button mushroom: 500 g	Walnut kernels: 20
Garlic: 16-20 cloves	Ginger: 1½ inches
Onion: 2 medium	Sesame seeds: 1 tbsp
Cloves: 4	Garam masala powder: ¼-½ tsp
Black pepper powder: ½ tsp	Rock salt: To taste
Curd: 2 tbsp	Water: 1500 ml
Sesame oil: 2 tbsp	

Method

1. Heat sesame oil in a pan. Add walnuts to it. Roast for 5 minutes or until they begin to change color. Remove walnuts from heat.

2. Roughly crush walnuts with the help of a pestle. Alternatively, grind 1 or 2 times in pulse mode. Do not grind walnuts to a fine powder, this will make walnuts bitter. Keep aside.

3. In the same oil, add sesame seeds and cloves. When they start crackling, add chopped ginger and garlic and cook for 2 minutes.

4. Add chopped onion and cook for 10 minutes.

5. Add sliced mushrooms. Cook for 5 minutes. Stir occasionally. Add rock salt and black pepper powder. Mix well and cook for 10 minutes. Take out 10 mushroom pieces for garnishing.

6. Add 250 ml of water and bring it to a boil. Simmer for 5 minutes.

7. When water is somewhat reduced, add another 250 ml of water. Bring it to a boil. Simmer for 5 minutes.

8. Turn the flame to low and add curd. Cook for 2-3 minutes.

9. Add another 250 ml of water. Bring it to a boil, then simmer for 5 minutes or until soup thickens.

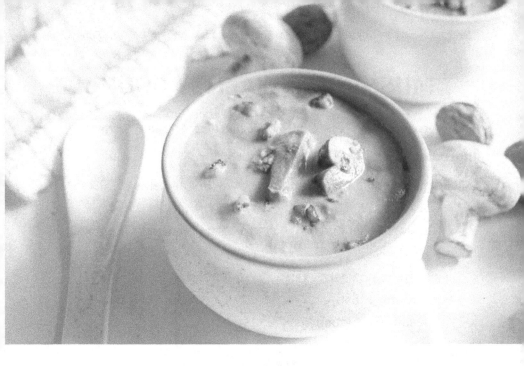

10. Add ¼ tsp of garam masala and 250 ml water. Repeat step 9.

11. Turn off the flame. Blend it into smooth soup in a blender. If required, add 250 to 300 ml of water while blending.

12. Bring the soup to heat. If the soup seems thick, add 200 ml of water. Taste and add ¼ tsp of garam masala if required. Bring it to a boil. Simmer for 5 minutes.

13. Turn off the flame. Pour soup in individual soup bowls. Add mushroom pieces and crushed walnuts. Mix and serve hot.

Tips

1. It is necessary to add water gradually to make the soup rich in flavor. Adding all the water at once will make the soup thinner and bland.

2. A total of 1500 ml of water was used for this soup. Your water quantity can range from 1300 ml to 1600 ml. So, add water gradually and adjust the amount of water as needed.

3. Over time, the soup becomes thick and strong flavored. If you are storing the soup for later, add 200 ml of water, adjust seasoning, and bring to a boil before serving.

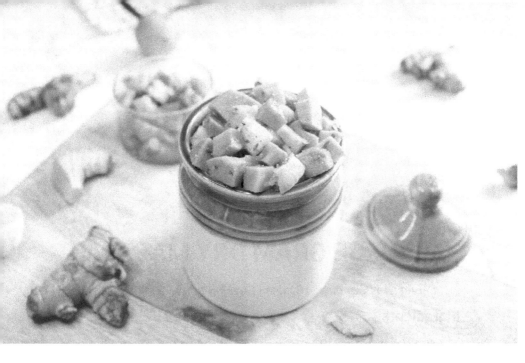

INSTANT TURMERIC PICKLE

Makes: 150 g | Prep time: 15 mins | Condiment

Ingredients

Fresh turmeric: 150 g	Lemon juice/Amla juice: 2 tbsp
Chopped Lemon: 2	Asafoetida: ½ tsp
Kala namak mix: 1 tbsp	Cumin seeds powder: ½ tbsp
Black pepper powder: ½ tsp	Mustard oil: 2 tbsp

Method

1. Wash turmeric thoroughly. Remove the skin. Finely chop them.

2. Add asafoetida, kala namak mix, cumin seeds powder, black pepper powder, mustard oil, and chopped lemon. Mix well.

3. Add lemon juice or amla juice. Mix well.

4. Spoon the mixture in a clean and dry glass jar. Cover the jar with a muslin cloth and keep it in sunlight for two days.

5. After two days, the turmeric pickle is ready to eat. You can store turmeric pickles in the refrigerator for up to 1 week.

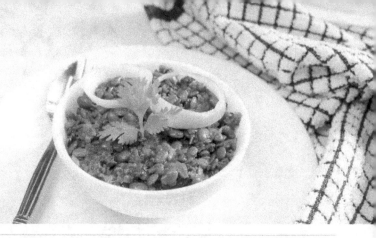

HORSE GRAM DRY MASALA

Serves: 4 | Prep time: 10 mins | Cooking time: 30 mins | Side dish

Ingredients

Horse gram: 200 g	Mustard seeds: ½ tsp
Asafoetida: ½ tsp	Cumin seeds: ½ tsp
Fenugreek seeds powder: ½ tsp	Onion: 1 medium
Tomato: 1 medium	Chopped Ginger-garlic: 1 tbsp
Green chilies: 2	Coriander powder: 1 tsp
Garam masala: ¼ tsp	Cumin powder: ½ tsp
Turmeric powder: ½ tsp	Bay leaf: 1
Water: 200 ml	Oil: 1 tbsp

Method

1. Soak horse gram overnight. Pressure cook horse gram with 200 ml water for 6 whistles. Grind onion, ginger, garlic, and green chilies with 2 tbsp water to make a thick and coarse paste. Grind tomatoes separately.

2. Heat oil in a pan. Add asafoetida, bay leaf, mustard seeds and cumin seeds. After a min, add onion paste. Cook for 7 mins.

3. Add tomatoes and salt. Cook for 5 minutes. Add fenugreek seeds powder, garam masala, turmeric powder, cumin powder and coriander powder. Cook for 5-7 minutes.

4. Add horse gram with stock and salt. Mix well. If necessary, add more water. Cover with a lid and cook on low flame for 15 minutes. Garnish with fresh coriander leaves and serve.

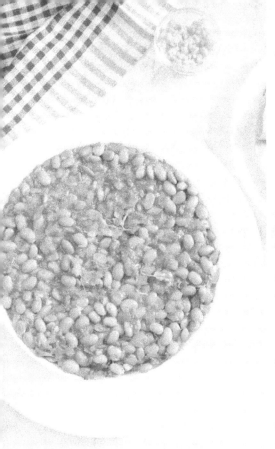

SOYBEAN MASALA

Ingredients

Soybean: 300 g	Onion: 4 medium
Tomato: 3 medium	Ginger: 1½ inches
Cloves: 3	Bay leaf: 1
Red chili powder: 1 tsp	Cumin seeds: ½ tsp
Turmeric powder: ½ tsp	Asafoetida: 1 tsp
Coriander powder: 1 tsp	Garlic: 10 cloves
Garam masala: 1 tsp	Salt: To taste
Coriander leaves: 1 tbsp	Water: 450 ml

Serves: 4 | Prep time: 10 mins Cooking time: 45 mins | Main course

Method

1. Soak soybeans in enough water overnight. Wash soybeans, pressure cook them with salt and 450 ml water for 5-7 whistles. Strain the soybeans. Keep the stock for later use.

2. Heat oil in a pressure cooker. Add asafoetida, cumin seeds, bay leaf, and cloves. Cook for a minute. Add chopped ginger and garlic. Cook for 2 minutes.

3. Add chopped onion. Cook for 10 minutes till the onions are tender. Add chopped tomatoes, salt and cook for 5 minutes.

4. Add turmeric powder, garam masala, coriander powder, and red chili powder. Mix well. Cover and cook on low flame for 10 minutes till the mixture starts releasing oil. Add soybean. Cook for 5-7 minutes. Add stock and pressure cook for 2 whistles.

5. Garnish with coriander leaves. Enjoy it with chapati and rice.

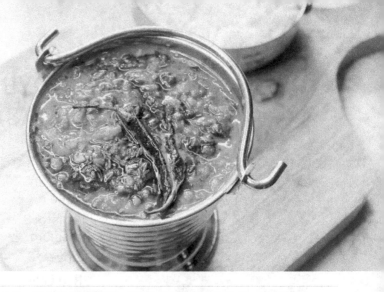

ROYAL HORSE GRAM DAL FRY

Serves: 4 | Prep time: 10 mins | Cooking time: 30 mins | Main course

Ingredients

Horse gram: 250 g	Garlic: 8-10 cloves
Ginger: 1½ inches	Onion: 3 medium
Tomato: 3 medium	Asafoetida: ¼ tsp
Cumin seeds: ½ tsp	Bay leaf: 1
Turmeric powder: ½ tsp	Garam masala: ½ tsp
Coriander powder: ½ tsp	Water: 800 ml
Red chili powder: ½ tsp	Salt: To taste

For Tadka

Dried red chili: 2	Kashmiri red chili powder: ¼
Asafoetida: ¼ tsp	Ghee: 1 tsp

Method

1. Soak horse gram overnight. Wash overnight soaked horse gram with fresh water and pressure cook with 500 ml water, salt, and turmeric powder on low-medium for 4 whistles.

2. Heat oil in a pan. Add asafoetida, bay leaf, and cumin seeds. Cook for a minute. Add ginger and garlic. Cook for a minute.

3. Add chopped onion. Cook for 10 minutes. Add chopped tomatoes and salt. Cover and cook for 10 minutes.

4. Add garam masala, coriander powder, red chili powder, and turmeric powder. Mix well. Cover and cook for 5 minutes.

5. Add horse gram along with stock and mix well. Add another 300 ml of water and bring it to a boil. Mash 30% of dal fry with a masher. Cook on medium flame for 5 minutes. Turn off the flame. Add tadka.

For Tadka

Add asafoetida, dried red chilies, and Kashmiri red chili powder to the hot ghee. Cook for 2 minutes. Add tadka to Royal Horse Gram Dal Fry. Serve with rice.

CABBAGE DRY FRUIT ROLL

Maeks: 18 rolls | Prep time: 20 mins | Cooking time: 40 mins | Dessert

Ingredients

Fresh cabbage: 1 large	Water: 500 ml
Jaggery: 80 g - 100 g	Licorice root: 2 inches
Clove: 3	

For Filling

Desiccated coconut: 60 g	Dates: 15 - 17
Walnut kernels: 4	Almonds: 10
Cashew nuts: 10	Pistachios: 10
Pumpkin seeds: 1 tbsp	Melon seeds: 1 tbsp
Rock salt: A pinch	Ghee: ½ tsp

Method

For Filling

1. Remove the seeds from the dates. Mash the dates with a masher to make them smooth. If the dates are not soft enough, beat them with a pestle to make them smooth.

2. Chop all nuts. Heat ghee in a pan and add all nuts and seeds. Roast till nuts start turning a little brown. Add desiccated coconut. Cook for 3-4 minutes.

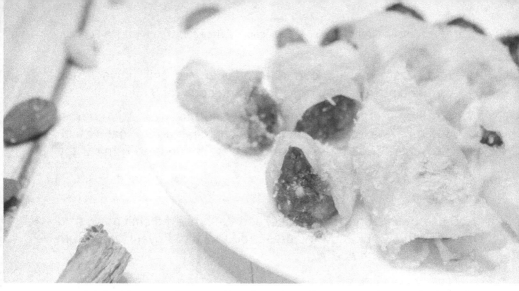

3. Add dates and a pinch of rock salt. Mix well. Cook for 2-3 minutes until the dates are soft and all ingredients are combined. Turn off flame and let it cool down for 5 minutes.

4. Grease your palm. Once the filling is cool enough to handle, make small laddoos. The laddoos need not be in perfect shape and should be slightly cylindrical in shape for easy rolling.

For Cabbage Roll

1. Wash the cabbage thoroughly. Remove the first hard layer of leaves. Make a horizontal cut at the bottom of the cabbage and carefully take out the cabbage leaves. Repeat the step to collect 9 cabbage leaves.

2. Put jaggery, licorice root, cloves, and water in a pan. Bring it to the boil. Simmer for 3-4 minutes.

3. When the syrup starts to thicken a bit, add cabbage leaves. Add 1 or 2 leaves at a time. Keep the flame on medium-high and cook for 5-8 minutes until the cabbage becomes soft and absorbs the flavor. Take out the cabbage from the syrup.

4. Repeat the process for all the cabbage leaves. Turn off the flame. Allow the cabbage to air dry for 2-3 minutes.

5. Cut the cabbage leaves vertically into two halves. If the leaves are too large, cut them into 3 pieces.

6. Place a laddoo at one end of the cabbage. Roll the cabbage. No need to seal the ends, when the cabbage will dry, the ends will stick together automatically. Make all cabbage rolls. Refrigerate for two hours and serve.

WALNUT CHOCO CHIA SEEDS PUDDING

Serves: 4 | Prep time: 40 mins | Cooking time: 10 mins | Dessert

Ingredients

Chia seeds: 10 tbsp	Milk: 1 L
Overnight soaked walnuts: 10	Cocoa powder: 3 tbsp
Honey: 2 tbsp or to taste	Licorice root: 2 inches
Cinnamon: 2 inches	Nutmeg: ½ small
Cashew nuts: 100 g	Water: 50 ml
Dry roasted walnuts: 2 tbsp	Chocolate shaving: 4 tbsp

Method

1. Soak cashew nuts in 50 ml hot water for 15 minutes. Blend cashews with stock to make a smooth cream. Refrigerate for 2 hours to set the cream.

2. Add cocoa powder, cinnamon, nutmeg, and licorice root to the milk. Bring it to a boil. Simmer for 5-7 minutes on low flame.

3. Turn off the flame. Cover and let it cool for 10 minutes. Remove cinnamon stick, nutmeg, and licorice root.

4. Add overnight soaked walnuts and blend until smooth. Take out the flavored milk in a bowl. Add chia seeds, honey and mix vigorously. Leave for 20 minutes to chia seeds to swell up.

5. Mix and break any lumps. Pour the pudding into individual jars. Chill in the refrigerator overnight or for 5-6 hours. Add cashew cream, chocolate shavings, roasted walnuts on top and serve.

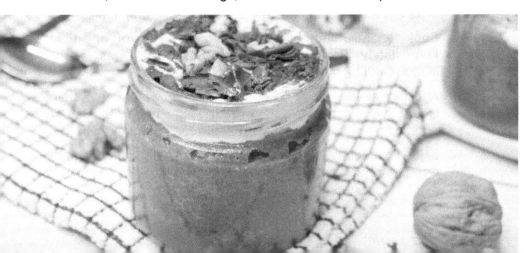

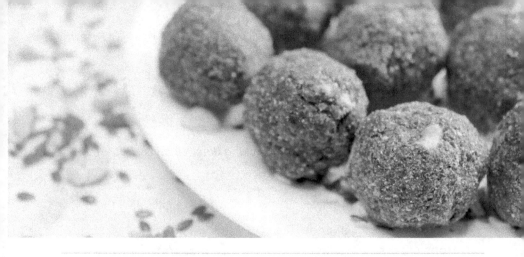

FLAX SEEDS LADDOO

Makes: 25 units | Prep time: 30 mins | Cooking time: 20 mins | Dessert

Ingredients

Flax seeds: 500 g	Cow's ghee: 2 tbsp
Chopped almonds: 100 g	Chopped walnuts: 100 g
Jaggery: 250 g	Tragacanth gum/gond: 100 g (optional)

Method

1. Dry roast the flax seeds on low flame till their color changes. Let the roasted flax seeds cool down and grind them in a grinder. Grate the jaggery and keep aside.

2. Heat ghee in a pan. Cook gond in the ghee till it swells. Take out the gond from the ghee. Let it cool and break it with a pestle or your hand.

3. Add nuts to the remaining ghee. Roast till they turn brown. Take out the nuts and add grated jaggery in same ghee.

4. Cook for 3-5 minutes till jaggery melts. Turn off the flame immediately. Don't cook jaggery after it dissolves, or else laddoos will be hard to chew.

5. Add flax seeds, nuts and gond. Mix well. Make round shape laddoo with hands while the mixture is still hot. If laddoos are not binding well, then heat the mixture for 2 minutes.

6. Enjoy Flax Seeds Laddoos. Store the remaining laddoos in the refrigerator and consume them within two weeks.

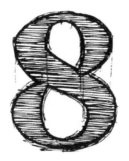

QUICK
SHORTIES

CARROT-WHITE RADISH INSTANT PICKLE

Chop 100 g carrot and 100 g radish. Add 1 tbsp panch phoran, 1 tbsp mustard oil, and ½ tbsp apple cider vinegar. Add salt and mix well. Eat with dal-rice.

GREEN GARLIC PICKLE

Chop 100 g green garlic and 2 green chilies and crush them in a mortar with a pestle. Similarly, crush 2 inches of ginger. Add 1 tsp mustard oil and salt to taste and mix well.

RAW PAPAYA CHUTNEY

Peel and grate 100 g raw papaya. Add salt, 1 tsp Kashmiri red chili powder, 1 tbsp brown sugar, ½ tsp coriander powder, and 1 tbsp extra virgin olive oil. Mix well.

ANTI-FLATULENCE CHURN

Dry roast 1 tsp carom seeds, 1 tsp fenugreek seeds, and ½ tsp asafoetida. Cool and grind them. Add black salt and mix well. Take half teaspoon of churn for belching and flatulence when required.

ARTHRITIS CHURN

Dry roast 50 g carom seeds, 25 g fenugreek seeds, and 5 g caraway. Grind them to make a coarse powder. Take half teaspoon of this churn with lukewarm water at night. Store the churn in an airtight container.

DIGESTION BOOSTER

Take a teaspoon each of coriander seeds, cumin seeds, and fennel. Soak them overnight in a glass of water. Drink this water in the morning to boost digestion in summer when required.

SPICY TOFFEE *(For cough and sore throat)*

Crush ginger (2 inches) and 10 black pepper. Add 10 g jaggery and 1 tsp cow ghee. Mix all ingredients and cook for 3 minutes. Take it as a toffee 2 times a day for cough and sore throat.

FENUGREEK WATER

Soak 1 tsp of fenugreek seeds in water overnight. Drink this fenugreek water in the morning on an empty stomach. Do it every day to control diabetes.

Thank you

Sign up to La Fonceur Newsletter to receive Bonus Recipes:

https://eatsowhat.com/signup

NOTE FROM LA FONCEUR

Dear Reader,

Thank you for reading *Eat to Prevent and Control Disease Collection (2 Books in 1)*. I hope you have found this book helpful. If you have a moment, please leave a review online. Help other health-conscious readers find this book by telling them why you enjoyed reading it.

Learn how a vegetarian diet is the solution to a disease-free healthy life in *Eat So What!* series- *Eat So What! The Power of Vegetarianism* and *Eat So What! Smart Ways to Stay Healthy*.

If you are looking for a permanent solution to your hair problems, read my book *Secret of Healthy Hair*.

All of my books are available in eBook, paperback, and hardcover editions.

Regards
La Fonceur

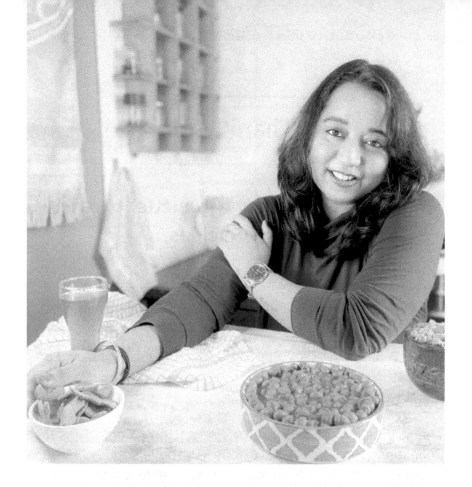

ABOUT THE AUTHOR

With a Master's degree in Pharmacy, the author La Fonceur is a research scientist and registered pharmacist. She specialized in Pharmaceutical Technology and worked as a research scientist in the pharmaceutical research and development department. She is a health blogger and a dance artist. Her previous books include **Eat to Prevent and Control Disease**, **Secret of Healthy Hair**, and **Eat So What!** series. Being a research scientist, she has worked closely with drugs and based on her experience, she believes that one can prevent most of the diseases with nutritious vegetarian foods and a healthy lifestyle.

READ MORE FROM LA FONCEUR

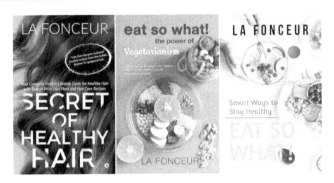

Hindi Editions

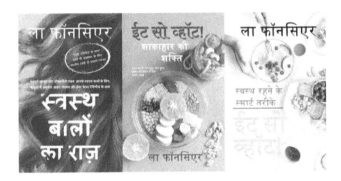

CONNECT WITH LA FONCEUR

Instagram: **@la_fonceur** | **@eatsowhat**

Facebook: **LaFonceur** | **eatsowhatblog**

Twitter: **@la_fonceur**

Follow on Bookbub: **@eatsowhat**

Sign up to get exclusive offers on La Fonceur books:

Blog: **www.eatsowhat.com/signup**

Website: **www.lafonceur.com/sign-up**